The Hard of Hearing Handbook

by
Caroline Bagshaw

IMPERIA BOOKS LIMITED

First published 1994
by Imperia Books Ltd.
© 1994 Caroline Bagshaw.

British Library Cataloguing
in Publication Data.
A catalogue record for this book
is available from the British Library.

IBSN 1 897656 05 X

Artwork by Mike Bagshaw
Cover by Sarah Davies
Typeset by Carter Wordsmiths, London

Published by
IMPERIA BOOKS LIMITED
Canada House, Blackburn Road, London NW6 1RZ

Printed in Great Britain by Black Bear Press Ltd., Cambridge

Foreword

By the Rt. Hon. Alfred Morris, AO, QSO, MP
formerly Minister for the Disabled.

This is an excellent book – and much overdue.

Approximately one in every six people in this country suffers from a degree of hearing loss. For some reason the hard of hearing are sometimes ridiculed by those with little understanding of the problem. As a result, their world can become bleak and lonely as they struggle to remain in contact with what is going on around them – but it doesn't have to be so!

This book does much to highlight the dozens of ways in which practical help can be made available – from hearing aids and the many other mechanical and electronic gadgets to hearing dogs and government grants. It shows how sometimes small adjustments can make huge differences to helping deaf people remain fully involved in all the processes of contemporary society.

The hard of hearing often find it a great strain to cope. The constant struggle to hear – what those more fortunate do naturally and without effort – can become deeply draining, both emotionally and physically. Another valuable lesson contained in the book is how such people can develop and then draw on their inner resources, and also on the help of others, to manage their emotions and renew their strength.

Almost equally important is the information the book brings to those who can hear – who mean well but are at a loss when attempting to talk to people with hearing disability. Public awareness has improved recently. You will probably have seen the ear logo (like the one on the cover of this book) in shop windows and other public places – which means the staff are aware of the problem and willing to help. But there is still a long way to go.

This book is essential reading for everyone with a deaf friend, acquaintance, colleague or member of the family – and that is almost all of us!

There cannot be a family in the country which does not have to confront this vexing condition at some time. The Hard of Hearing Handbook deserves a place on the bookshelf in every home.

Alf Morris

Contents

Preface

Chapter 1 **What Is It Like Being Hard of Hearing?**............1

What is it like? Misunderstandings. Why don't they wear hearing aids? Lipreading problems. Tinnitus.

Chapter 2 **Psychology Matters** 15

Recognising the problem. What to do. Helping yourself. Your attitude. Psychology of coping. Emotional reactions. Stress.

Chapter 3 **How To Communicate**............33

How do you communicate? Learning to lipread. Golden rules for you. Golden rules for those who want to be heard. Other methods of communicating.

Chapter 4 **Hearing Aids** 55

Types of hearing aid. Special features. Getting the aid. Learning to use the aid. Care of the aid. Looking after the aid. Problems. NHS or private? Comparison of services.

Chapter 5 **More Technical Help**............72

Alarm clocks. Doorbells. Smoke detectors. Microphone pick-ups. Television. Loop system. Telephone. Out and about. Prices and availability.

Chapter 6 **Outside Help, Problems at Work & Public Awareness**....84

Social services. Employment. Public awareness.

Chapter 7 **Hearing Dogs** 98

Sponsorship. Selection. Socialisers. Training. How to get a hearing dog. What if you don't qualify?

Chapter 8 **Deafness and the Ear**............106

How the ear works. Types of deafness. Causes of deafness. Hopes for the future.

Useful Addresses............117

Preface

I'm thirsty.
It's not Thursday.
I know. Could I have some water?
Some what?
Water.
What for?
I'm thirsty.
So what if it is Thursday?

And so it goes on. Comic it may be, but it is a confounded nuisance for everyone. It is a nuisance having to repeat things and to find things not done on the grounds that someone did not know what was said. But it is far more of a nuisance to those who are struggling to hear, constantly wondering if they have got it right and anxious about how many times they can reasonably ask again.

Deafness is a little understood handicap because it is invisible. Nothing happens to the ears – at least not to the outside bit you can see. They do not shrivel or droop. You only know that people are finding it hard to hear if they say so.

The obvious signs, like misunderstanding and a confused expression, are associated with low intelligence. So the deaf are patronised. Maybe people do not realise they are doing it. They just assume the deaf cannot join in – so they just do not include them, except now and then.

Despite appearances, deaf people are every bit as able as everyone else. If you find that hard to believe, stuff your fingers into your ears. Has your intelligence dropped?

It is hearing, or rather not hearing, that causes all the problems. So it makes sense to do everything possible to make hearing as easy as possible. There are all sorts of ways of doing this, both high-tech and low-tech. That is what this book is about.

Chapter 1
What Is It Like Being Hard of Hearing?

For the purposes of this book, "deaf" means having a hearing loss that causes problems – whether slight problems occasionally, or severe problems frequently. "Hard of hearing" and "hearing-impaired" have the same meaning.

How many?

There are 7,500,000 hearing-impaired people in the UK.

Of these, some 300,000 have such a severe impairment that speech, even in the best of circumstances, is hard to decipher. Most of them still rely on speech to communicate with others, using lipreading, pen and paper, and helpful friends. There are about 50,000 who prefer sign language. Their thriving friendship circles of "signers" are known as the deaf community; and they lead lives as rich and full as do the rest of us.

The remaining 7,200,000 have a mild to moderate loss. Not even audiologists agree exactly what these terms mean. It is hard to be precise anyway, since hearing depends on so many things – as, for example, how much background noise there is or whether someone is speaking from behind a newspaper. A mild to moderate loss means that a person can hear quite a lot if the conditions are right – but not nearly so much when conditions are unfavourable.

What is it like?

It is in the nature of things that the hard of hearing find it difficult to communicate.

It is not surprising that many hearing people have no idea what it is like. They imagine a hushed world where shrieks are like whispers, and rush-hour traffic like a babbling brook. If only it were that simple!

There is a type of deafness in which all sound is muffled. This suggests a simple blockage – such as wax, or pus from an infection – that is preventing sound waves from getting through. That sort of deafness is usually easy to treat or much improved by a hearing aid.

Most deafness is more complicated. The commonest cause is damage deep inside the ear. Sound waves bounce along until they reach the inner ear, where they should get translated into recognisable sounds like words, music or whatever. But this does not happen as it should if the inner ear is damaged. The brain then receives distorted signals, which it interprets as distorted sounds.

Some signals do not get sent at all – so there is no sound heard. Others come through quietly. Others, believe it or not, come out over-loud. The end result is a jumble of quiet, loud, and distorted noises with bits missing. No wonder the hard of hearing find the effort of trying to listen so exhausting.

Distortion

Poor quality announcements at railway stations come close to imitating what it is like to be deaf. Many people complain that they cannot hear these announcements but they do not mean that at all. What they hear is loud enough; but the actual words are lost in the general crackling and distortion. It is like that all the time for deaf people.

Another way of illustrating this is to put a radio out of tune. You can still hear words but find it difficult to follow them. Turning up the volume just makes it worse. It has a similar effect on the deaf when well-meaning people start shouting.

Recruitment

Recruitment, when an audiologist says it, has nothing to do with looking for people to do a job. It means loudness discomfort.

When sound reaches a certain volume it becomes uncomfortable. A little louder still, and it hurts. It is like that for hearing people too – but for them it takes something like a pneumatic drill to cause pain. For a deaf person, walking along a busy road might have the same effect.

It may seem strange if a deaf person complains of too much noise when a hearing friend does not. It has to do with making proper sense of the sound, rather than detecting it.

Inside the inner ear are thousands of microscopic hairs that move in response to sound waves. They cannot move so subtly if they are damaged; but then they can over-stimulate the nerve fibres leading to the brain –

resulting in more noise for a deaf person than for a hearing one.

Beethoven was a classic example. When war reached Vienna in 1809, nobody much cared for the noise of gunfire but Beethoven could not stand it at all. He fled to his cellar and remained there, clutching cushions over his ears, until the battle was over.

Recruitment makes background noise a big problem. It does not have to be gunfire. The gentle hum of machinery might make other hearing impossible for the deaf, especially when the higher frequencies are lost. Background noise tends to be of a lower frequency than speech – so it is often heard more clearly.

Cocktail party deafness

Cocktail party deafness is the name given to problems with the background noise encountered at cocktail parties or gatherings where several conversations are going on at once.

Some people, who can hear perfectly well most of the time, find hearing difficult when there is a babble of voices in the background. This may be a first sign that their hearing is beginning to deteriorate.

Willis Paracusis

The condition is named after Thomas Willis, the seventeenth century doctor who first described it. Willis told the story of a deaf lady who could only hear in the presence of a din. Her husband regularly employed a drummer to provide the noise necessary to enable them to talk to each other.

People who suffer from Willis Paracusis have the opposite problem to those with cocktail party deafness. They need background noise to stimulate their ears into working.

It has been suggested that the din does not help the hearing as such but makes people speak up. That cannot be the whole story or drum bands would be a cure for deafness – which they most certainly are not. The loud noise probably gets the bones inside the ear moving; and then the quieter sounds are simply carried along with the loud ones.

Location of sound

Two ears, equally good or equally bad, are needed to tell where sound is coming from. The ear nearer to the sound source will find it slightly louder than the one further away. So if it sounds louder in the right ear, the sound is coming from the right. If in doubt, moving the head soon gives a good idea.

This does not work if one ear is better than the other. All sound will seem to come from the better side. If one ear is a lot better than the other, it may be impossible to tell where the sound is coming from.

People who locate sound easily take this ability so much for granted that they do not realise how difficult it is for those who cannot.

One lady was irritated to discover her teenage son had gone out and left his music on full blast. Try as she might, she could not find which of the myriad of knobs was the off-switch. Frantic, she went to a neighbour for help. He stopped the noise at once. It was not coming from the music centre at all but from a tape recorder on a different shelf.

Another lady left her baby with a hearing-impaired baby sitter for the first time. She felt anxious and phoned home to check that all was well. The sitter heard the phone but could not find it. So the worried mother rushed back to find out why nobody was in.

Hearing aids may help with this – but probably not. Sound heard through a hearing aid has a different quality to that heard naturally. It is difficult enough to hear at all with a hearing aid without also having to make special judgements.

People can help by saying where they are when they call out – such as "I'm behind you" or "I'm in the living room". Most people just say "I'm here", which is no use at all.

How misunderstandings arise

Granny isn't really deaf. She just puts it on sometimes. It's really embarrassing. I took her to my office the other day. When my colleague said "How are you?" she was all smiles and it was fine – so she heard that all right. Then she suddenly started saying "Pardon?" all the time. Sometimes she didn't answer at all. I ask you! She can hear well enough when she wants to.

It makes Granny sound unreasonable; but it is far more likely that she is deaf. Not totally deaf, but deaf enough to cause problems – one of which is that people like her grandson do not understand her difficulty.

There are people who seem to think that you never hear anything if you claim to be deaf. And also that you must be able to hear everything if you do hear sometimes.

But hearing is not like that. Nobody can claim never to have said "What was that?" Deaf people have to say it very much more often.

What happened to Granny at the office was a typical experience for the hard of hearing. She had wanted to be friendly and make a good impression. Whether or not she heard the "How are you?" does not much matter. It is very likely that someone shaking your hand and smiling is saying that or something similar – and the response is easy. It was more of a struggle after that.

What her grandson did not notice was that the photocopier had been switched on just before his grandmother suddenly started saying "Pardon?"; and that this background noise had drowned out his voice. He also did not realise that his colleague had turned his head away when his grandmother did not answer; and that she did not even know he had spoken. It is to be hoped that the colleague had more understanding than the grandson.

Understanding is important. People feel hurt and cross when they think they are being ignored and they blame the person who is ignoring them. The excuse of deafness seems hollow when it appears to vary from minute to minute. It is important to appreciate that it only looks like that because of constantly changing background conditions, such as the noise of photocopiers and the position of a speaker's head.

Background noise

Hearing people may think that background noise is not a problem for the deaf because, being deaf, they cannot hear it. But some noises are heard better than others; and speech is not necessarily the best. Hearing people are also better at filtering out unwanted noise.

There is a limit. In a really noisy place, like an iron foundry or a nightclub, no one can hear normal speech. So sometimes people say to the hard of hearing "It's just as bad for me when there's a lot of noise".

But there is a big difference in the amount of background noise needed to make conversation impossible. For the deaf, a busy cafe can have the same effect as a nightclub for the hearing. The general buzz of voices in the cafe, along with the noise of crockery and cutlery, can take on monster proportions for the hard of hearing and make it exhausting even to try to listen to a conversation. The result is often a grimace; and that may be why deaf people are constantly being told to cheer up.

Recruitment

Recruitment, as mentioned above, means loudness discomfort.

For many deaf people, there is little difference between too quiet and too loud. They may complain that they cannot hear the television. But when it is turned up, they say that it sounds horribly loud and uncomfortable – and they still cannot hear it. This generates impatience. "She just wants to be awkward!"

A normally hearing person can experience something like this by turning up the volume to very loud indeed. There comes a point when it is annoyingly loud. Depending on the quality of the television, it may be distorted as well. For people suffering from recruitment, the level above which discomfort is caused is very low – not much above muffled.

This means that shouting is not helpful. It does nothing to make the voice clearer and it tends to fluster the deaf person, who does not know what is being said but can tell from the wide open mouth that the person is shouting. Nobody likes being shouted at. So the deaf person becomes defensive and the other, who meant to help, thinks "ungrateful so-and-so" and gives up.

Vowels and consonants

People with good hearing assume that speech comes at an even level of sound, with every letter at the same volume as every other. This is not so.

The sound level of normal speech rises and falls all the time. The difference between the strongest sound (aw) and the weakest (th) is about 30 decibels. It is true that the voice can be raised and lowered to make the sound even; but this does not happen in natural speech.

The vowel sounds come out louder. That is why they are used to attract attention. "Oi!" can be sustained in a loud voice. People use consonants if they want to attract attention quietly. "Psst!" It would not be possible to say "psst" loudly enough to make someone hear at a distance, for the sound dies away as the mouth opens wide.

This is of no importance to hearing people for they hear consonants with perfect ease and the fact that they hear vowels even more easily makes no difference. But deaf people may hear vowels quite easily while having difficulty with consonants.

This is another reason why shouting does not help. It brings out the vowels at the expense of the consonants. It is quite likely that the vowels were heard the first time – but they did not make sense without the consonants.

Unfortunately, it is the consonants that are needed to make speech intelligible. Speech would still be decipherable if vowels were abolished. Hearing only vowels makes communication very difficult.

Try to understand this well-known quotation with the consonants taken out.

.a.. a.. .i.. .e.. u. ..e .i..

If that is too difficult, try shouting it. Does that make it any easier? Try the same quotation again, this time with just the consonants.

J.ck .nd J.ll w.nt .p th. h.ll.

The chances are that you got it immediately. It would make life much easier for the hard of hearing if those who can hear would realise how much more important it is to enunciate clearly than to shout.

Change in conditions

People with good hearing have plenty to spare. They can be in different rooms, with the television on and the clattering of pots and pans around them, but still hear each other talking.

This makes it hard for some to believe that the sound of a voice can be obliterated for a deaf person just by moving a few feet further away. They may scoff "It didn't make any difference. It sounded just as loud to me". But if they actually measured the sound, they would find that its volume had been reduced to one quarter of what it was by moving from one metre away to two metres away.

Take a situation in which two people are sitting opposite each other at an empty table in a well-lit quiet room. These are near ideal conditions. lipreading is at its easiest. The sound is coming straight from person to person and there are no distractions, visible or audible. Most deaf people will cope with that. So a hearing person will be deluded into thinking all is well.

But suppose he gets up, walks across the room, looks out of the window and then speaks. Conditions seem nearly enough the same to him – but to the deaf person, the change is drastic. He is likely to hear little or nothing.

Depending on the distance from table to window, the sound volume could be a tenth or less than it was before. The sound waves, instead of coming direct, hit the window first and then scatter. Also, lipreading has become impossible as the face is no longer visible.

Why don't they just wear hearing aids?

There are a lot of misconceptions about hearing aids. People think that, just as spectacles can transform blurry blobs into sharp outlines in an instant, hearing aids will bring immediate, crystal-clear hearing.

Short-sightedness is an altogether different situation in which the lens of the eye is not working properly. Putting an artificial lens of the right shape in front of the eye corrects the defect – resulting in normal vision.

Hearing aids do not bring normal hearing or anything like it. What they do, basically, is to make everything louder. This would be fine if all sounds were equally difficult to hear – but that is far from the truth.

The usual situation is that low-pitched noises, such as traffic, are easy to hear. In fact, that sort of noise intrudes. With a hearing aid they intrude even more. It is possible to ignore them with time and practice. But it is so unpleasant having unwanted noises amplified, and such hard work trying to blot them out, that many people just give up.

It is possible to get more refined hearing aids (see chapter 4) but these are rarely available on the National Health Service; and even the most sophisticated will not restore normal hearing.

Hearing aids are most effective when the problem is a simple blockage that prevents sound from getting through – but that sort of deafness is easier to treat anyway.

About 80% of deafness is caused by damage to cells deep inside the ear, making it difficult for the brain to interpret what comes through to it. No hearing aid can mend these cells. So, with a hearing aid, the hotchpotch of confused noise that is the result of deafness comes through just the same – but louder! It takes a lot of patience to learn to use a hearing aid effectively.

There are still problems, even when people persevere and learn to pick out the sounds they want by concentrated practice. Any sudden change in the level of sound, such as a dog beginning to bark, may make the amplified sound intolerable – so they turn off the hearing aid. Sometimes, they forget to switch it on again, causing great hilarity when this is discovered. "She's deaf but she doesn't even turn on her hearing aid!"

Another problem is that nearby sounds are amplified more effectively than sounds coming from further away. This is fine if the nearby sounds are the wanted ones – but that is not always so.

There was a lady with a fairly new hearing aid who thought she was doing rather well. She was able to attend meetings and one triumphant day, when the secretary was ill, she was asked to take the minutes. It was an effort to hear the man at the far end of the table but she managed it. Then the person sitting next to her tore a sheet of paper off a pad. Its sound drowned out the more distant voice.

"I'm sorry," she said. "I didn't get that." "Pull the other one," was the rude reply. "You can't just suddenly stop hearing." In vain she explained that the sound of paper tearing had drowned out his voice. Nobody else had even heard it. How could she, being deaf, have known about it? They thought she was putting it on.

It must be understood that aided hearing is very different from natural hearing. Too many people think that hearing aids solve all problems.

Lipreading problems

Lipreading is a great crutch for the deaf but it is by no means a perfect substitute for hearing.

Same shape – different sound

Lips move a good deal when talking; but most of the sound is made further back, inside the mouth, throat, nose and lungs. Many quite different sounds have similar lip shapes, like "t," "d" and "n".

Take one example. "Read" and "drink" sound very different but look alike, especially when preceded by "to". It is not always obvious where one word ends and another begins. "To" is often slurred over, pronounced as a simple "t," which looks the same as "d". This can easily be attached to the "r" of "read" and so be interpreted as "dr". "Ea" and "i" have the same basic shape, so "to rea-" can easily become "to dri". "D" and "n" also look alike, so "read" becomes "drin". "K" is an invisible sound, so its absence will not be noticed.

If someone thinks he has been asked "Would you like something to drin," he is likely to assume a "k" is there. Then, if what the hostess actually asked was whether he would like something to read in bed, he may feel put out at having to go back to the kitchen to make a cup of tea. Unless she knows about lipreading, she is likely to think he is just being demanding.

The need for a clear view of the mouth

Lip movements are unimportant to those who can hear, so they do not bother to keep their mouths clearly visible. They tend to look away if something distracts them or if they are thinking hard. If they are talking about a picture behind them, for example, they may well turn to look at the picture as they speak. Then they are surprised that the deaf person has missed bits of the conversation but still heard some things. "He hears if he can be bothered", they conclude to themselves.

Objects can easily obstruct the view of the mouth – fingers, cups, pens, sheets of paper. Even movements near the mouth, like stroking the chin or rubbing the nose, can be distracting. So too are bushy beards. Cigarettes and chewing gum are by far the worst for they prevent the lips from moving intelligibly.

A retired vicar once got the wrong idea because of a cigarette. He thought a smart young man had asked the way to the cathedral. What the man had actually said was "casino." Both words begin with the same letter, have the same rhythm and nearly the same vowel sounds. The differences between "s" and "th," and "o" and "al" are difficult to discern from lips that are holding a cigarette in place.

Tinnitus

What is it?

Everybody gets tinnitus – those noises in the ear after bonfire night and similar noisy events. For most, it goes as suddenly as it comes. For some, it goes on and on... and on forever.

The dictionary describes it as "ringing, hissing or booming." That is correct but it does not stop there. It also buzzes, pounds, throbs – you name it and someone, somewhere, has tinnitus like it.

Living with constant noise is tough and some people are driven to despair. Van Gogh may have been one of them. It is not known why he cut off his ear but many tinnitus sufferers have got hold of their ears in a frenzy, as though to yank them off. Alas, it would make no difference if they did, one way or the other.

Although it "drives you mad" in the sense of making you cross and fed up, tinnitus has nothing to do with real madness. Some people panic, thinking it is the beginning of the "voices" heard by some psychiatric patients. That worry can be discarded immediately. Tinnitus makes just about every noise known to man; but it never, ever, gives instructions to go out and do the work of God or of the devil.

Where does it come from?

Nobody knows for sure exactly what tinnitus is. The Ancients thought it was caused by minute animals setting up home in the ear. You can understand why when you hear it.

We do not know much more today. Tinnitus is sometimes called a phantom noise. The theory is that the auditory nerve, although deafened, does not shut up shop. Its job is to transport sound, in the form of electrical impulses, to the brain. If real sound stops coming through, it then manufactures its own – tinnitus.

This is compared to the phantom limb of an amputee. When a limb is lost, the nerves that used to lead to the missing part go on sending signals; and the patient gets the sensation that the limb is still there. It could be that the auditory nerve also sends out phantom signals.

Another theory is that tinnitus consists simply of body noises like breathing, heartbeat, blood flow, etc. These processes are far from silent as any stethoscope will reveal. We do not normally hear them because there are always other, louder noises. There are noises everywhere – muffled traffic sounds, faint gurgles from the plumbing, and so on. Body noises come to the fore when people stop hearing these others.

Whether these theories are right or wrong, one thing is agreed – tinnitus is a terrible nuisance.

What can be done about it?

The usual advice is to learn to live with it. There is as yet no cure. Research for this non-dangerous condition is starved of funds and gets only about

2p per sufferer per year from the government.

Even with unlimited funds it is difficult to research something that cannot be seen in any way, shape or form. No microscope, x-ray or scanning machine has yet shown tinnitus in action.

Some forms of tinnitus have a simple cure, so it is worth consulting the GP about it. There could be too much wax in the ear or the sufferer may have taken too many aspirins recently. At the other extreme, there is a remote possibility of its being a symptom of something more serious.

By far the most likely outcome is that the doctor will say "This is not dangerous in any way but I can't do anything about it." That does not mean there is nothing you can do. There are lots of tricks you can try.

Distraction

You stop noticing the tinnitus when you are thoroughly absorbed in some activity. This may be hard to believe when the tinnitus is so insistent that you find it hard to concentrate on anything else. But doing what you enjoy most does make this possible. So you need to enjoy yourself as much as you can. This is pleasanter advice than "Just put up with it".

Enjoyment is effective because it makes you concentrate on something else. Any activity that requires concentration can help, including dull ones like attending to your paperwork. There is no limit to the possibilities – jigsaw puzzles, learning a craft, rock climbing, etc.

Listening to it

Some people go the opposite way. They actually listen to their tinnitus, think about it, analyse it and try to predict what it will do next. Then it becomes an absorbing occupation in itself. This works for some; but for others, because it is essentially dull, the attention soon wanders.

Smetana, the musician, did more than just listen to it – he composed a piece of music based on it (the final movement of his first string quartet in E minor). This could be excellent therapy for someone with musical skills. The composer can exercise a degree of control over the tinnitus and communicate what it is like. Most of us, sadly, cannot communicate in that way.

Story telling

This is something that can work when you are trying to get to sleep. Use the tinnitus noise as a background to a story. If it is a waterfall, imagine yourself walking beside it. Feel the spray on your face and the sun on your back. Get out the picnic hamper. If it is a steam train, make it the Orient Express. Climb aboard. Order dinner. Tell the other passengers your life story.

Your imagination need not be brilliant but just good enough to set your mind on another train of thought – anything but tinnitus!

Old wives' tales

Old wives' tales can be wise tales containing ancient wisdom. They are still resorted to when doctors can offer no obvious remedy for some ailment.

Since there are always new problems, there are always new wives' tales and tinnitus has created hundreds. It does not matter if your doctor turns his nose up at them. If they work, they work. Steer clear of experimenting with pills and potions, starving yourself, or undertaking tough exercise routines, as then, at least, you will come to no harm. The following have all worked for someone.

- Glucose drinks on waking.
- Strawberry tea.
- Carrots, cut into sticks – one stick every half hour or so.
- Cider vinegar, liberally sprinkled on meals.
- Pineapple juice with meals.
- Muesli at bedtime.
- Pressing behind the ears with fingers.
- Pulling the ear lobes gently round in circles.
- Massaging the face.
- Long hot bubbly bath – peering out over the bubbles, imagining it is a snowscape while basking in the warmth.

Drowning it out

Some tinnitus is so piercing and persistent that it is the loudest noise around.

Most sufferers are more fortunate than that. They do not notice it when they are busy – for everyday noises are sufficient to drown it out. But it returns just as soon as things become quiet.

The natural reaction is to make a noise, any noise, to drown it out. So people start humming, turn on the radio or get out the Hoover. Periods of rest are ruled by the need to make a noise.

Rather than be robbed of your rest periods, you can plan what noise to have. Listening to a tape is more relaxing than pushing a Hoover up and down. Any tape you like, music or stories, will do. There are tapes made specifically for the purpose (contact the Royal National Institute for the Deaf or the British Tinnitus Association – see address list). There are recordings of natural environmental sounds like waves breaking on the beach. Or you can record any sound you find soothing. If the Hoover is the right pitch, make a recording of that. Ignore the guffaws. Only you know what is best for you.

Maskers

There are devices called maskers, specifically designed to drown out tinnitus. Some fit in the ear. Others go on the bedside table to help you to sleep. They mostly make a shushing noise called pink noise. For some people, they are the solution.

You may be able to obtain one on the NHS. If not, they cost from about £50 to £600. The British Tinnitus Association (see address list) provides extensive information.

Acupuncture

There is some evidence that acupuncture can help to relieve tinnitus.

The effect seems to be only temporary; but it works again if the treatment is repeated. Practitioners are easy to find. Acupuncture is sometimes provided at conventional health centres. Otherwise consult the Yellow Pages.

Chapter 2
Psychology Matters

Recognising the problem

Most deafness creeps up slowly. Hearing goes from good to not quite so good without anyone noticing. People can manage very well with slightly substandard hearing. Then it gets a little worse, and so on until one day it becomes a problem. But since it is only just a little worse than it was a short time ago, people often fail to realise what has happened. They just notice the effects. "Dad's a proper grump these days" they conclude.

It may well have occurred to Dad that he does not always hear; but if he is like most people, he will have shut out the thought. He does not want to be deaf. Clearly he is not completely deaf; so he denies that he is deaf at all.

This creates more problems than it solves. Everyone thinks that everyone else is being awkward. "I told him. Why didn't he listen?" goes up the cry. "But she never said. How was I supposed to know?" he snaps back.

Then a row breaks out about whatever happened because he did not listen/she never said. Tempers erupt because library books were not returned or potatoes not bought. Members of the family dwell at length on library fines or on only having sandwiches for dinner. It is all a million miles from "Give me a few seconds and I will hear you."

Why don't people recognise it?

Deafness is a special disability because it brings blame down on the sufferers. Deaf ears look exactly like hearing ears. It is not possible to tell who is deaf by looking. A lot of the signs like looking vacant, or taking no notice, are also signs of low intelligence or stand-offishness. And, as often as not, that is how they are interpreted.

A man out on a bitter winter's day, and wearing a woolly hat with ear muffs and a heavy hood, will not hear much. When he pulls it all away from his ear and says "What?", it is accepted that he did not hear and that is the only reason for his slowness. He is unlikely to be called "cloth-ears" despite the layers of cloth that did cover his ears. But that same taunt may well be made to someone else with uncovered, normal looking ears who says "What?". He gives the impression that he is not too bright.

No one is more acutely aware of this than the deaf themselves. Being with a group of nodding and smiling people, and only knowing vaguely what they are talking about, is daunting. Saying "Excuse me, I'm deaf" takes nearly as much courage as saying "Excuse me, I'm daft".

The natural reaction is to bluff through and to nod and smile with them. Venturing a comment is like sticking a foot out over the edge of a precipice. People may carry on talking or they may suddenly stop and look. You do not know until you try.

All this makes social contact frightening. Some people avoid socialising altogether rather than face it. Some try to hide it by chattering constantly – that gets them out of trying to listen. Some become aggressive and blame everybody else for not making things clear. Many, who are thought of as unsociable grouse-pots, are not naturally like that at all. They have been made so by the experience of deafness.

Experimental deafness

An experiment was carried out in which volunteers had their ears plugged with wax and cotton wool for twenty-four hours. That did not stop them from talking to people if they concentrated; but it did prevent the easy flow of general conversation.

Twenty-four hours is not long to induce a personality change but the volunteers felt that that was what was happening. Being deprived of the simple chit-chat they had always taken for granted made them want to run away. They felt more than embarrassed by not being able to follow conversations – they felt rejected! Some felt the words they could not hear must be directed against them. Their self-confidence slumped and they began to avoid people. It was a hard day and they were thoroughly bad-tempered by the end of it.

They all knew that their deafness would be totally cured on the following day. How much worse it is for those who fear – many with good reason – that it will last for ever.

What to do

The first step is to go to a GP who will examine your ears. The problem could be caused by a simple build up of wax that can quickly be syringed away, or by an infection treatable with antibiotics.

If the GP cannot find a simple way to restore your hearing, you will be referred to an Ear Nose and Throat (ENT) clinic. There you will be seen by a specialist and be given hearing tests. Perhaps you may also have other tests, such as X-rays, depending on what the problem is thought to be.

Hearing tests

There is a wide range of hearing tests, from whispering at you with your eyes shut, to connecting you to a computer that measures the activity of the auditory nerve. The usual tests involve listening to a series of sounds through headphones.

The first time can be a dispiriting experience. You are led into a small soundproof chamber and the door is shut behind you. This is where the truth will be revealed. Isolation hits hard.

The test is simple. You are given headphones and told to indicate when you hear a sound, usually by pressing a button. At first you will hear easily but eventually there comes a point when the sound is very faint. Did you hear something? You are not sure. Do you press the button? If you do and there was no sound, you might look a fool. But if you do not and there was a sound, you will give the impression that your hearing is worse than it is.

The answer is "Yes, you should press the button if you think there may have been a sound". People with normal hearing are also unsure about very quiet sounds; and the tests allow for some error.

The results will be written up on a special graph called an audiogram. That represents your personal hearing loss, shown as a series of circles, crosses and lines. It looks pretty meaningless to the uninitiated but gives a good deal of information to the trained eye – not just about the hearing loss but about the likely cause and the best way to proceed.

Hearing aids

If you are lucky, the doctor will suggest some way of improving your hearing. This might involve an operation. Mostly though, there is no appropriate treatment other than supplying a hearing aid.

Unfortunately, it has to be said that most hearing aids are a disappointment – at least at first. Many people think it will be like switching the ears back on; but reality is so different that the bulk of hearing aids are put away in a drawer and forgotten. One survey suggested that of all hearing aids issued, only half are still in use a year later and only 3% are used regularly.

This is a shame because hearing aids, used well, can make the world of difference. It is a matter of allowing sufficient time and being prepared to learn how to use them, slowly and patiently.

It is easiest to start practising with someone whose voice you know well, one to one in a quiet room, and only for half an hour at a time. You can then progress gradually to using the hearing aid with several strangers and in noisier surroundings.

Some people wear their hearing aids all day, every day, and feel lost without them. Others take theirs off for a rest from time to time. Thousands of people do benefit. Probably, with proper training, millions more could.

Hearing therapists

Hearing therapists come in at the point when the hearing aid is first fitted.

They help the patient adapt to using the aid and also give information about available equipment and about the patient's other requirements. Their knowledge covers the social, educational, vocational, medical and technical needs of the hearing-impaired. So a hearing therapist should be able to answer all the patient's questions or advise who else to ask.

Unfortunately, although the DSS first recommended the use of hearing therapists in 1975, there are still not enough to go round and not everybody can be offered the service.

In some districts the gap is plugged to some extent by volunteers. You can enquire whether there are "befriending" schemes in your area. These are usually manned by people who have successfully conquered their own hearing aid problems and understand what a struggle this can be.

Speech therapists

Many deaf people fear that their speech will become incomprehensible. This is extremely unlikely.

Most people who suffer in this way have been profoundly deaf since they were babies. They have never heard speech and so cannot imitate and learn to use it.

People who learn to speak before they lose their hearing are almost certain to retain their speech as normal. The only exceptions to this are people who become so deaf that they cannot hear their own voices and so cannot monitor them. Even in these cases, speech therapists can help.

Former MP, Jack Ashley, is a prime example of someone who, although severely deaf for 25 years, has never lost his clear diction.

Helping yourself

People often get caught in a vicious circle. Not being able to hear upsets them – so they become aloof or else tend to snap back when approached. This irritates others, who are less likely to be helpful as a result. So the deaf person gets more upset, more aloof and more bad-tempered. The others back off even more. And so on... and so on.

It is possible to break out of this; but it does require effort. The deaf person has to push forward, constantly seeking help along the way. With help, communication becomes easier and this is an encouragement to talk and listen more. Other people will respond better and that brings more encouragement, more confidence and more friendship. We all enjoy friendship, whether deaf or not.

Sometimes it will not be too difficult to cope. Some people speak ever so clearly and some rooms have good acoustics. You can kid yourself for quite a time – but the longer you do so, the longer it will be before you start adjusting to your loss.

The first step forward is to accept your poor hearing as a fact and to agree that not everyone around you is suffering from laryngitis! This is a tough one.

Enlisting the help of others

You should not try to cope on your own. You need to tell other people. Those close to you probably at least half realise it already.

They may have been through the same "I wonder if... I don't really think... Yes, I do think so" process that you have. It is much easier once it is out in the open. Then you can all talk about what you need to do.

Telling new people is more difficult. There is often one first embarrassing moment of revelation; but most people will be glad to help. Human beings are gregarious on the whole and want to be thought friendly. If they seem distant at first, it may be because they too feel embarrassed and do not know how to be helpful.

Occasionally, you may meet a pathetic creature who thinks it's fun to sneer at disability – someone who keeps saying "Eh?" in a loud voice, and laughing. You can forget that person without a qualm. Don't let it put you off meeting others.

However willing, people cannot help if they do not know how. A typical reaction of the well-meaning is to shout – which is worse than useless. It distorts the sound, changes the shape of the mouth and looks unfriendly. But you cannot blame people for not knowing. You need to tell them.

It is not necessary to deliver a lecture – just a pointer or two:
It's easier if you look at me when speaking. Would you mind talking just a bit slower?

Self-help groups

Even the most sympathetic family and friends will become bored with discussing your hearing problem long before you do. Even if they never complain, you may begin to feel a little guilty about burdening them.

Self-help groups provide the best support for people with a common problem. Those in the same boat talk about their troubles more avidly than anyone else. Talking about it again and again, round and round, is just what they need.

Other people who share your problem need to talk endlessly about it, just as much as you. You will perform a useful service by listening and by chipping in with your bit. You can feel virtuous too for being willing to help others with sympathy and advice.

A hard of hearing club may already exist in your area. You can find out by asking at the library or at the Citizen's Advice Bureau. Or you can contact one of the national organisations for the deaf (see address list).

If there is no convenient club available, you could write a letter to the local newspaper asking if anyone would be interested in starting one. Since one in six of its readership is likely to be hard of hearing too, you should get a good response.

What affects how well you will cope?

It might be thought that the greater your hearing loss, the worse your life will be. But that does not necessarily follow. Two people with identical audiograms might lead completely different lives, one ruined and the other fulfilled.

Perseverance

Beethoven had become completely deaf by the age of forty-nine, long before many of his greatest masterpieces were composed. You might take a leaf out of his book. For a musician to lose his ability to hear music could have been devastating – but Beethoven was determined to conquer it.

One of the many things he did was to make himself a sort of hearing aid out of a piece of wood. He put one end on the piano and the other in his mouth. That sent vibrations through his teeth. From this and his memory, he could sense what the music sounded like.

It is not a solution that immediately leaps to mind; but Beethoven kept on thinking and trying. Music was his life and he was not going to give it up because he could no longer hear.

You do not have to be good at music to learn from this lesson. Go for whatever it is you want to do! Refuse to be discouraged!

Expectations

One big difference between Beethoven and those who sit at home sobbing is in what they expect from life.

People with an optimistic outlook will thrust themselves forward. If something does not work, they will shrug their shoulders and try again. If a recommended piece of equipment turns out not to be right for them, they will take it back and try another... and another... confident that in the end they will find something good – and they will.

Pessimistic people hide away. If one outing is unsatisfactory they will be reluctant to try again. They do not expect much of any equipment. When the first flick of the switch does not bring crystal clarity, it will confirm to them that nothing works. So they will try nothing else and get nowhere.

Optimists and pessimists both get what they expect. Their attitudes are self-fulfilling.

Think positive

There is a solution out there somewhere. There is a vast array of technical equipment (see chapter 4) and all sorts of useful tips from other sufferers. With so many millions hard of hearing, there are bound to be plenty of ingenious ideas.

To give just one example, during World War II there was a deaf man who lived alone and found that the air raid sirens did not wake him. These days he could have a sound-sensitive system linked to a vibrating pad under his pillow – but not then. Instead he had a long piece of string. At bedtime he tied one end around his wrist and threaded the other end through the window, so that it dangled down to the pavement. Everyone knew what it was. When the sirens sounded, the first person who passed gave it a tug and up he got.

That man had something in common with Beethoven. He spent time thinking about what he could do – rather than about what he could not.

Your attitude

How you see deaf people

It will be hard for you to come to acknowledge your own difficulties if you think that deaf people are somehow inferior.

Some people deliberately seek out difficult situations in order to prove they are not handicapped. They may insist on playing Trivial Pursuit when they would enjoy Patience more. You can play Trivial Pursuit if you want to – but be sure it is Trivial Pursuit that attracts you and not the opportunity to prove a point. You are not a failure if you opt for Patience, or gardening, or silent movies, or any of the scores of quiet hobbies that can be enjoyed by people with any level of hearing.

How you see yourself

Your self-image can have a big impact on your ability to cope. If you see yourself as a victim, you are likely to waste much time and energy in resentment. Your energy is better spent in thinking of yourself as someone with a task to perform – to be able to communicate fully with others despite the obstruction of rotten hearing.

If you see yourself as a hearing person gone wrong, you will strive too hard to prove you are as good as the others. Extra help directed to you will then seem like a sly dig, drawing attention to your inadequacies.

Instead, see yourself as a different sort of person – different in one way and one way only. Then you may expect to be valued in the same way as everyone else. You will interpret any help given to you as recognition of your worth.

The challenge

There is no need for loss of hearing to be thought of as a calamity. It is bound to bring difficulties; but thinking that things are impossible can only make them worse.

Seeing it as a challenge, as something that demands exploration, will lead on to better things. Exploration opens up new avenues, new experiences and new fulfilment.

One lady discovered this after finding she could no longer hear the bingo numbers being called. Her friends missed the next number when they tried to help her – so she had to give up bingo. She was upset at first but took up chess, rather than sit at home moping. To her surprise, she found that she had a gift for it. It brought her new friends, new prestige and a new interest.

She had gone through the same horror and fears as most deaf people. But with time, thought, effort and lots of support, she found that, in one way, her deafness had done her some good.

Crying over spilt milk

Deafness is better faced square on. If you cannot get rid of it, you just have to live with it. So, you need to think calmly about how deafness is affecting your life and what you can do to change those effects.

It does you no good to moan about not being able to watch a video. Go to the library and borrow a copy with subtitles. That will put you back with the hearing crowd and you will no longer need to moan.

Having said that, it is tiring constantly having to think of ways around difficulties. It is far easier just being able to listen. Now and again you may need to cry over spilt milk. Do so. Nobody can be brave, strong and resolute all the time.

A few tears, a bit of moping and the odd yowl of protest "Why me?" can renew your strength for the battle ahead. Self pity is only destructive when it becomes a way of life.

So, if it sometimes seems all too much, retreat. Cry, moan, say "It isn't fair" (it isn't!). Then go back, think about what you have to do, and start doing it.

The psychology of coping

Given time, most people reach the stage where they do not mind too much about being deaf. That is bad if it means they have given up. One way of coping is to pretend that it does not matter – to hide away and avoid anything that involves hearing. This may seem like making the best of a bad job but it is not getting the best out of life.

It is normal to feel like giving up in the early stages of deafness. Jack Ashley did, saying "I have no future". But he was wrong. He continued in his chosen career and excelled. So have thousands of others.

Most people go through a predictable pattern of behaviour as they gradually come to terms with being deaf and begin to build their lives around that inescapable fact.

I'm not deaf. I'm not. I'm not

People resist bad news and seek ways of explaining it away. This is easy with gradual deafness and they can go on for years like this:

Children aren't taught to speak clearly these days. I've got a bad cold today.

It is more difficult with sudden deafness – but people try all the same. They tell each other stories about someone who was deaf for a week and then walked into a lamp-post and was cured. Sudden deafness does sometimes cure itself; and so people go on denying that it is permanent for as long as they choose.

A man who had fallen off some scaffolding was told there was little hope for his hearing. He spent a depressing afternoon straining to hear a mowing machine through the open hospital window. It seemed silent. That night he dreamt that his ears were full of grass cuttings and the doctor was applying the tube of a vacuum cleaner to his ear. He had half accepted that there was no cure in reality; but his subconscious mind was still looking for one in fantasy.

24

I'm not deaf, but...

Problems begin to get noticed but they can still be explained away. If a phone call was slow and difficult, perhaps it was a bad line. If the alarm clock was not heard, perhaps it did not go off. But suspicions arise when things like that keep on happening.

Deafness affects different people in different ways. A man may still be able to use the phone easily while his wife is quite unable to do so. But she can hear the birds singing when her husband hears nothing. Each can claim to have better hearing than the other, and so affirm that it is the other who is deaf.

I'm deaf. Everything is ruined

It finally comes to the crunch. At some point deafness creates real problems. Perhaps an attempt to buy something has to be abandoned because the sales assistant seems to be miming. Or a favourite television programme is switched off because it is just too hard to hear it. Something happens that makes the deafness impossible to deny.

Time to panic. Suddenly, instead of there being no problems, life is nothing but problems. They can't do this and they can't do that. Any suggested solutions are parried with a "Yes, but..."

You could get videos with subtitles.
Yes, but subtitles get in the way.
You can get special phones.
Yes, but I like the phone I've got.

This is the halfway stage. The sufferers have accepted that there are problems – but making use of items designed for the deaf is going too far. They still cling to the idea that they can hear really.

They are still in grief. Everywhere around them people are talking and listening. There seems no way of ever joining in again. The deaf retreat and brood about being left out. It seems that this phase will last for ever.

I'm deaf. I must do something about it

The urge to communicate is so strong that people usually keep on trying. With support, they find that they can communicate – at least for part of the time. This spurs them on to try again and to hunt for more solutions.

Fifteen-year-old James was nonplussed when his grandmother asked to borrow his Walkman. It was her vigorous complaints about his music that had made him use it instead of his stereo whenever she visited the house. But she had not become a pop fan. She had been thinking things through.

She knew that James could hear things through his Walkman that no one else could; and she wondered whether it could help her. It did. She could hear the sound clearly when it came straight from the radio to her ear – even though she had given up trying to hear it from across the room.

She switched off the rock music quickly. Then a broad smile spread over her face as she tuned in to a tape of The Archers. She had entered the phase of taking positive action – the beginning of renewed self-confidence.

Being deaf is part of me

This is a stage of triumph. No more brooding on the loss of hearing, for there is happiness ahead.

Plans are made for the future as eagerly as before. Any problems that deafness brings are dealt with – but not dwelt on. It has even been known for people to say that if a cure were found they wouldn't bother with it. They cope perfectly well, thank you.

Most do have lingering regrets; but their lives are now too full of other interests to spend much time thinking about them. People do not progress smoothly from one phase to the next. There are bleak days in which they trudge backwards into gloom, and bright days when they skip forward again. Back and forth they go.

But overall, there is a regular path along which most people travel. First comes shock and denial. This is followed in turn by realisation and despair. Finally, they reach the stage of taking stock and coming to terms with their disability.

Getting stuck

Sometimes people get stuck at an early stage. They just go on denying or despairing.

Some denial and some despair is to be expected. All aspects of the loss must be thought through before things can be put into perspective. But if this goes on and on, months turning into years, it will get progressively more difficult to make progress.

It may then take a conscious effort or jolt to start nudging forward. This is far easier to do if you understand fully what is happening.

Emotional reactions

The typical feelings experienced by people struggling to accept that their hearing is deteriorating are anger, fear, and a sense of loss.

Anger

To the deaf it seems grossly unfair to be no longer able to do something as natural as hearing. And, make no mistake, it is unfair!

Loss of hearing makes difficulties in situations that should be perfectly simple – like finding out whether a cardigan is available in a different size. People become angry and get fed up when this sort of thing keeps on happening.

Some begin to treat such situations as tests. If they do not catch what is said, they have failed the test – or the other person has failed. A minor mishap becomes a personal failure.

There are scores of opportunities to set up tests like this each day. Every time it does not quite work, more anger is generated against themselves or against other people.

They cannot accept that some adjustment is essential, some mistakes inevitable. They build a brick wall against which to bang their heads.

Fear

People worry, quite reasonably, about how they will cope. This can escalate into real dread when people assume the worst.

They know nothing of lipreading, hearing aids or any of the 200 plus assistive devices on offer. They assume that nothing can be done. Helpful suggestions are rejected out of hand.

I can't lipread.
I tried that once.
Hearing aids are useless.
I can't understand technical things, like loops.

They fear that they will not be able to cope, even with a lot of help.

Rather than face that prospect, they refuse all help. It can be more comfortable to wallow in the misery of hopelessness than to try hard and fail.

But they still worry; and their worry leads them into a situation in which they have even more to fear.

Sense of loss

A degree of loss is inevitable; but some people feel they have lost everything. They refuse to think about what they can do – but only about what they can't. One bad thought leads to another, on and on, down and down, until they sink into an imaginary catastrophe.

I used to be the life and soul of committee meetings. Now I'm not even certain what they're saying. I think I got it right about how they're changing procedure; but suppose I haven't? ...

I might be doing it wrong. We'll lose the business ...

I'll get the sack. I won't be able to pay the mortgage ...

This is called catastrophising. Thinking about real loss and the possible consequences encourages the imagination to run riot. That gets in the way of doing something positive about it. So things may well really get worse.

Dwelling too much on the loss may lead to more loss in the end.

Crooked thinking

Being deaf is not the end of the world. If you think it is, that is probably because you are in an emotional state and are not thinking straight.

What you need to do – and it is not easy – is to step outside yourself and take a long cool look at how you are thinking. Very likely, you've got it crooked.

It is time to talk to yourself. It is not a sign of madness, and you need not talk out loud. But when you start thinking that life is impossible, ask yourself three questions.

Am I brickwalling?

Brickwalling means banging your head against a brick wall of your own making. People often do this when they yearn for something they cannot have.

If that something is acute hearing, they may for example blunder through a phone call and be too proud to accept help. Then they become defensive and use words like "must" and "can't", "always" and "never".

I must always make my own phone calls. I'll never have one of those funny phones.

This attitude allows no room for changes, even changes that would improve the quality of life. Think about it if you catch yourself saying that things have to stay the same. Turn your statement into a question and ask why. This can open up a path to a better future.

Why must I always make my own phone calls. Wouldn't it be easier if someone else listened, and relayed the message to me?

Why shouldn't I have one of those funny phones. It might look better than my old-fashioned thing.

Am I making assumptions?

When things are going badly, people tend to start assuming that they will get steadily worse. It is difficult to try again if someone has an embarrassing encounter and then creeps away without putting it right.

It's club night, but can I go? I'm still reeling from last week when John asked me if I'd watched the play on Sunday and I went and washed the plates. They were all laughing when I came back. Then he asked me again and I realised. I'm a laughing stock. I won't go.

In this case you can ask "What is the evidence for that?" Often, there isn't much. Did those people know she had misheard? Perhaps they assumed she thought it was time to wash the plates. What were they laughing at? It could have been anything. Even if they did know, why should they think ill of her? Perhaps John felt bad because he had unwittingly sent her to do a chore.

Am I catastrophising?

People get on to a run of bad thoughts. Starting with a reasonable fear like "My hearing may get worse", they helter-skelter into despair – "I will be stone deaf soon".

The question to ask then is "What is the worst I can really expect?" The answer is that your hearing probably will get worse. Virtually everybody's does in time – but it is a slow process that gives you time to adjust and look around for solutions. Meanwhile research is going on and the outlook may be much brighter in five years time.

Another question to ask yourself is "Suppose the worst really does happen. What can I do then?" The answer is "Lots". Pretend for a few minutes that you can hear nothing at all. There is still hope. The chances are that a cochlear implant will help. You can practise lipreading. You can have a textphone. You can apply for a hearing dog. And so on... and so on.

Fewer than one percent of people with a hearing loss are profoundly deaf. You are most unlikely to join them. If you do, there is lots that can still be done. Many profoundly deaf people lead rich and exciting lives.

How to stop bad thoughts

The best way to stop a chain of unpleasant thoughts is simply to say "STOP" – even out loud if you are on your own.

Then fill your head with something trivial. Recite the alphabet backwards. Learn your 17 times table. It does not matter what you do – so long as it has no connection with your problems and is difficult enough to make you concentrate.

This should clear your head of nasty thoughts. Once they are safely banished, the way will be clear to think about the good things in your life.

You can make thinking good thoughts a definite aim. The vague "Things are OK really" will not help. You need specific thoughts about things that are going right. These need not be huge – small blessings will fit the bill very well.

Even though it's a nuisance waiting in the clinic for two hours, I do get my knitting done ...

Now that I can hardly hear the television, I do a lot of reading. I never realised there were so many good books ...

I get just as much joy out of gardening. Hearing, or not, makes no difference.

Reactions to stress

When you feel stressed, your heart pounds, you breathe faster and your muscles tense up. This is a deeply ingrained reaction that dates from the time when stress meant being faced with a sabre-toothed tiger.

Then, as now, the body instantly prepared itself for fight or flight. Breathing speeded up to get in extra oxygen, the heart raced to pump the blood round, and muscles tightened to gather strength to club the tiger or to flee for dear life.

Sabre-toothed tigers have gone but the stress response remains. The body reacts in the same way to alarming situations, whatever the cause. You know that a group of chattering people will not sink their teeth into you; but the fear they may look askance may be enough to affect your heartbeat, breathing and muscle tension.

It works the other way round too. The fact that you are breathing hard makes you feel afraid. Your tense muscles make you feel tense.

Even if you can do nothing about the basic situation, you can still improve the effect it has on you by controlling your breathing and relaxing your muscles.

Breathing exercises

Breathing exercises can be done anywhere and at any time, even in front of strangers – they need never know.

Your body is demanding extra oxygen. Give it some by taking one deep breath. Then let the air out slowly, thinking "Calm down". After that, take long, slow breaths. Breathe in. Hold it for a short time – long enough to feel in control but not long enough to feel uncomfortable. Breathe out slowly.

Do this a few times and then breathe normally. Don't do it continuously. You can repeat the exercise later if you still feel out of control.

Relaxation technique

The technique of relaxation is simple. First you make yourself comfortable, lying or sitting in a warm room with your arms by your side and your legs slightly apart. You can be perfectly quiet or you can put on some background music. Music is better if silence brings out your tinnitus.

Then, taking different groups of muscles in turn, first tense them and then relax them. The usual way is to begin with the feet and to go on to the calves, thighs, buttocks, stomach, shoulders and face. The order is not vital; but it is easier to remember if you go from one end of your body to the other. There are tapes you can buy if you wish to do it to a set pattern.

For each group of muscles, you tense up and hold them like that – making yourself aware of what it feels like. Then you relax – noticing the sensation of the tension ebbing away.

Repeat the process with the next set of muscles. And so on, until you have worked through all the muscle groups. The session ends with a few minutes of total relaxation before slowly getting up and returning to everyday life. It may seem odd that relaxation exercises involve first tightening the muscles as much as you can. The idea behind it is to learn to recognise the difference between a tense muscle and a relaxed one.

You may think that is obvious – but it isn't always. Many people are tensed up all day long without ever realising it. They then wonder why they feel so tired when they have done so little. Tensing muscles is hard work.

A problem you may encounter is that other muscles tend to follow suit when one tenses up. Try tensing all the muscles in your face by making a horrible grimace. Your shoulders will probably hunch at the same time and your stomach will harden and your fists begin to clench.

That makes sense when you realise that tension is a primitive response to threat. It has to be all or nothing. It is no good having hard fists and floppy legs when the sabre-toothed tiger threatens. We have not changed so very much since those primitive times and we still tense all over when we feel threatened – even when the threat is only of embarrassment.

Relaxation sessions teach you to recognise quickly when your muscles are tensing and to enable you to relax them. Some of the mental tension disappears with the physical tension. You are in better control. Your body becomes more relaxed and so does your mind.

Chapter 3
How To Communicate

How do you communicate when you can't hear?

Lipreading

Watching lip movements is another way of understanding the words if you cannot hear them properly.

It is not a perfect way, despite those crime novels that would have you believe that a detective can follow a conversation at any distance with a pair of binoculars. Unfortunately for Interpol, there is no hope of that. The detective might think he'd discovered that the jewels were in the petrol tank, when what the crook actually said was "The shoes are in the bedroom, Hank". If you do not believe that could happen, try it for yourself in front of a mirror.

Lip movements are only a small part of the total mechanism of speech. In medical textbooks, diagrams of the organs of speech show the lungs, the throat, mouth, nose, an amazing amount of tongue and the lips. Sound is made by air being pushed around the various parts and out through the mouth or nose. Moving the lips is just one part of the process.

Some lip shapes are shared by different sounds as there are not enough shapes to cover all the sounds. Some lips are lazy and hardly move at all. Ventriloquists have tuned this to a fine art – yet people still manage to understand the dummy with its one and only mechanical mouth movement. This might seem discouraging. If lip movements have so little effect, how can lipreading help?

But lip movements are important. Ventriloquists sacrifice clear speech in their act. Those sounds that cannot be said with stationary lips are replaced by something else. "I oo-ant sung discuits, klease" says the dummy; and the audience immediately understands "I want some biscuits, please." A lot of help is also given by the story line.

This should encourage up and coming lipreaders (who might be any age up to 100 or even beyond), as it shows how people can still understand when the lips are not as helpful as they might be.

Lipreading is called "Speechreading" in America because it is recognised that watching the lips is only one aspect of the skill, which also involves facial expression, body language, general observation, information about the subject and listening. This may sound complicated; but it is only an expression of what people do naturally without thinking.

Facial expression

The expression on a person's face tells you the sort of words he or she is likely to use. If it is disapproving, it is more probable that "ugly" rather than "lovely" was said. If it is confident, "cheering" is a better bet than "jeering".

You need not worry about learning lists of possible words. The human brain is excellent at categorising and automatically discards the improbable.

So this is one lipreading skill you already possess.

Body language

The way we stand, sit, lean, hold our heads and so on, says a lot about how we are feeling. This is called body language.

It is not an exact science. You cannot look up someone's posture in a body language dictionary and know all their secrets – but it can be telling. A lifeguard who yells "Get out" at boys playing raucous ducking games in the swimming pool may not be heard – but the boys will know what he said.

You can sometimes use body language to predict the likely trend of a conversation. If you see a friend slouched against the wall and looking down, he is probably dejected. If he is moving around, smiling and giving little jumps, you can deduce that he is happy. If you know that he has just taken his driving test, you will expect him either to talk about the iniquities of test examiners, or about the driving trips he is planning to make.

Observation

Even when two words look similar on the lips, you can often guess from the context which one is being pronounced.

For example, the words "paper" and "baby" look the same on the lips but they are not often interchangeable in a sentence. A visitor to a new mother, holding a furry bunny, is unlikely to open the conversation with "Where's the paper?"; whereas a woman with a pen in her hand, opening and shutting drawers, is unlikely to be asking "Where's the baby?"

It could happen that a brand new grandmother, expecting a visit from the new arrival, is also conducting a running battle with the paper boy. She might say "The baby came today" or equally, "The paper came today" with the same look of triumph.

In that case, the thing to do is to ask "Did you say paper?" or "Did you say baby?" If you ask "Did you say paper or baby?" she will repeat the word and it will still look the same, leaving you none the wiser. Ask one or the other for a "Yes" or "No" answer. Fortunately, "Yes" and "No" look nothing like each other on the lips. "Yuh" and "Nuh" might be confused though – so speaking clearly is important.

Information

It is easier to follow a conversation if you know something about the subject matter.

People can sometimes gabble on without actually saying what they are talking about.

I went up to town because that's the best place, and I got one. But when I got home, it wasn't the right sort – but it still might work if I can get the other one.

That sort of speech makes you spend energy in trying to work out whether you have missed something and, if so, what? You are unable to concentrate on the words; and so you may miss the key word, if it ever comes.

It is much easier when people state the subject matter at the beginning.

About my holiday – I went on a railway tour. All the trains were late on the first day.

About that building site. They're working very fast. All the drains were laid on the first day.

"T" and "d" have similar mouth shapes, so "train" and "drain" or "late" and "laid" could easily be confused. But knowing whether the subject matter is holidays or building sites makes it obvious which was said.

It also depends on how much you know about the subject. A computer buff will recognise the word "megabyte" immediately; whereas someone for whom a computer is just a weird magical box will be at a complete loss. "Mud pies" perhaps?

It is difficult to recognise the names of people to whom you are introduced when you have been given no prior information. A name might be anything. Some are very similar to each other in lip shape – like "Meryl" and "Beryl," and "Kevin" and "Gavin". You might even get the gender wrong with names like "Cheryl" and "Gerald". But the names of people you know, especially your own name, will be easy because they are so familiar.

Listening

Few people are completely deaf; and you should use to the full what hearing you do have – with or without a hearing aid.

Some people see lipreading as a test. They think they are not proper lipreaders if they lipread a bit and also hear a bit at the same time. But lipreading is not just lip watching. It is a way of communicating by using all available means, including listening.

Spelling

English is a rich language, having had bits added to it from all the country's invaders and visitors since the year dot. This has made its spelling rich, or ridiculous, depending how you look at it.

To take just one example, the sound "sh" can be spelt sh, as in shop; ch, as in machine; ti, as in attention; si, as in tension; ss, as in pressure; ci, as in precious; ce, as in ocean; or xi, as in anxious.

Pages could be filled with examples of the varied spellings of single sounds but they make not one jot of difference to the spoken word. The same sound makes the same lip shape, however it is spelt.

We are so familiar with the written word that spelling can sometimes get in the way. For example, if someone is talking about giraffes, the lipreader might just get the "j" and "f" sounds, and start searching through the memory bank for something like "j*f*" and come up with "jaffa". Giraffe does not come readily to mind because the sound "j" is so firmly associated with the letter "j" that one forgets it can also be spelt with a "g".

So, when lipreading, try to forget everything you know about spelling.

Learning to lipread

The best way of learning to lipread is to do it.

Everyone can – at least a little. Small secrets are mouthed behind people's backs. Nightclubs are so noisy that any talk there might just as well be mimed. And there are lots of other situations like these.

Learning to lipread means building on skills you already have – and not starting from scratch.

Classes

Many people are reluctant to go to classes because the idea smacks of school. Memories of bad schooldays may linger on; but the atmosphere in a lipreading class could not be more different. There is no talk of detention or visits to the headmaster. It is more like a social club with learning and benefit thrown in as a bonus.

You do not need to be a great scholar. Learning the technical details of every sound and lip shape will not necessarily make you a better lipreader. You need only learn to associate the lip shape you see with the sound you would hear if you could. The best way of doing that is to practise.

You can practise by looking carefully at people's mouths when they talk to you. This will help you to improve. But you will progress faster and better if you go to a class. There you will be taken through the sounds in a systematic way and be given lots of practice with specially designed material. You will also meet people in the same boat as yourself. There will be much talk about hearing problems and how to solve them. You are far more likely to stick at it if you are part of a group of friendly people than if you struggle on alone.

Another advantage of a class is that it gives you the chance to practise being assertive in sympathetic conditions. If your failure to understand makes you a nuisance, that will be accepted. It will also be accepted that you will go on being a nuisance until you do understand.

You will be with people who know exactly what it is like and will help you when you flounder. They will flounder too; and you will all get help from each other and eventually stop floundering. Being one of many will stop you feeling stupid; and that will stand you in good stead when you need to ask for help in ordinary situations.

Lipreading classes are widely available at adult education centres. Many of them are subsidised and some are free. Enquire at the library, at the office of the local education authority or at the audiology clinic.

Practice

You will need plenty of practice whether or not you go to classes.

Most of this will be in real conversations as you go about your normal business. But you can also set aside a special time if you know someone willing to sit and practise with you. It matters little whether or not your partner hears well.

There are other ways of practising if you find this too embarrassing or if there is no one available to help.

In front of the mirror

You can study your own lip movements in front of the mirror.

The advantage of this is that you can do it at odd moments during the day – say when you are getting ready to go out. Little and often is not a bad way to learn.

The disadvantage is that, as you know what you intend to say, you will not know whether or not you are learning to distinguish the lip shapes well.

It is also better to have a variety of faces to practise with, rather than just your own. Mouths do vary. There are thick lips and thin lips, lazy lips, mobile lips and lips surrounded by assorted beards and moustaches. You will only see one sort in the mirror.

Television

Though television is sometimes suggested as a ready source of people talking, it is far from ideal for lipreading practice.

Programmes are produced for dramatic effect and not for clear views of mouths. There are distant shots as well as back views and close-ups of people listening to others talking off-screen. And if there is something in front of an actor's mouth, there is nothing you will be able to do about it.

A boy and girl were making tentative advances towards each other in a romantic scene at a bus stop. The camera moved slowly from one to the other as they talked. From time to time, the pole of the bus stop obstructed one mouth or the other. Hearing people did not notice; but for the hard of hearing the effect was as if the romantic couple had hiccups. Every now and then, their words suddenly became garbled.

News programmes are better. Newsreaders are selected for their ability to speak clearly. You get a clear view of the face and there is often a picture behind to help. For example, with a picture of a house half under water, you know that the subject matter is floods. On the other hand, newsreaders give very little away in facial expression or body language.

Another problem is that people tend to turn the volume off in the misguided belief that it would defeat the purpose of the practice if they hear anything. There is no reason why people with little hearing should try to manage without it. They should always use whatever hearing they have.

Some people are so discouraged by unsuccessful attempts to lipread the television that they decide they just can't lipread – and give up. This is a pity. Though lipreading may sometimes seems impossible, it really is a great boon.

One way of using the television for lipreading practice is to follow the subtitles. This is not cheating. You need more information than just lip movements – and in the real world you get it.

Subtitles will not show precisely what the people are saying; but they come close. You will recognise the spoken words – not all, but some. Each one you recognise is one more success in associating a lip shape with a sound. Also, you are learning to use the additional information that is available – which is an important part of lipreading. And, even if your lipreading skills are temporarily at low ebb, you may enjoy the programme.

Keep at it

Don't be discouraged though it may sometimes seem impossible to get any meaning at all. It will come more readily at other times. The more you practise the easier it will become.

Early researchers called it "ocular audition" – which is a high-flown way of saying "hearing with the eyes". That is a good description because, at its best, lipreading gives the illusion of hearing.

Causes of confusion

Unfortunately "hearing with your eyes" is something you can only keep up in short bursts. If every sound had a distinct lip shape all of its own, looking would be as good as listening. As it is, lots of sounds share similar lip shapes – and some have barely any shape at all.

You only have to get one sound wrong to get the wrong end of the stick completely. For example, the phrase "braying for justice" conjures up an image of a lynch mob demanding instant retribution. "Praying for justice" sounds more like people on their knees, quietly imploring the Almighty to make the right decision. That is an easy mistake to make, as "p" and "b" look exactly the same when spoken. "M" is in the same group. So "the monks were praying for justice" might be heard as "the punks were braying for justice" – which sets a different scene altogether. This creates false expectations for the rest of the story, which is likely to get more and more confused.

You stand a better chance of avoiding this sort of situation if you know which sounds most often get confused. Then if the word seems wrong, you can try substituting another one you know looks similar. That might make more sense. There are many examples of these and I will give just a few.

Sh, Ch, J

Did she get the job, or did he get the chop? Either way makes the same mouth shape – though it should be easy to tell which from her facial expression.

Facial expression can give you a guide as to whether you are getting it right. A man in a pub was surprised when the barman said he was going to give his wife a "right shiner" for her birthday. He seemed happy about it and not at all annoyed. It became clear later that the planned present was "white china".

S, Z, X

The most famous example of this confusion is when Nelson, mortally wounded in the Battle of Trafalgar, was heard to say "Kiss me, Hardy". He may have done; but it is far more likely that he said "kismet", meaning this was his fate. The "s" in "kismet" is pronounced "z". Nelson, on the point of death, would have spoken quietly and his crew would have lipread rather than heard. "Kiss me" made a better story – so it stuck.

The "x" sound is pronounced "ks" however it is spelt. As "k" is difficult to see, "x" is often mistaken for "s". One man was puzzled when told about a woman who "did a lot of good worse". What on earth could it mean? She was actually a charity worker who did "good works". The final sound of "works" is "x", despite the spelling.

"X" is also confused with "z", which is also occasionally spelt with an "x" as in "xylophone". Mostly it is spelt with a "z" as in "zoo", or "s" as in "wise". Whichever it is, it is the pronunciation that counts and not the spelling.

A mother rebuked her mechanic son when he came round without his tools. He had promised, she said, to mend her car. He claimed not to have said anything like that – but to her, he had. He had promised to come and "visit". She thought he said "fix it".

T, D, N

"Her house is really tiny. I don't know how she manages it because it's a huge house". This apparent contradiction makes perfect sense when you substitute the "n" of "tiny" with a "d" – making "tidy".

The confusion between "d" and "n" can make the deaf seem colour blind. If they are sent to get a green ticket, they may well come back with a red one. "G" is a difficult sound to see. If it is missed, the word seems to start with "r". Knowing it is a colour is likely to lead to the assumption that it is red. The "n" at the end confirms that, as it looks just like "d".

K, G, Ng, Nk

Words like pick, pig, ping and pink, or rack, rag, rang and rank, look the same as each other on the lips. Someone you think got stung in the leg may actually have got stuck in the lake. If you are wondering why someone wants some string, it could be that they want a drink.

P, B, M

"There's a mop in the kitchen", the woman thought she heard her husband say when she came home from shopping.

"Why didn't you put it away, then?" she thought crossly. When she got to the kitchen, she found a group of hungry schoolchildren. Her daughter had invited her friends home and was busy emptying the fridge. The man had said "mob" not "mop".

Sometimes, the change of sound makes little difference. It does not matter whether someone is "making" or "baking" a cake. "Bad" and "mad" may in effect mean much the same. But there is a lot of difference between a "pink coat" and a "mink coat", or "shooting rabbits" and "shooting rapids".

Vowels

The vowel sounds are less important than the consonants in shaping a word. They differ anyway with different accents – something that has to be coped with by deaf and hearing people alike.

Clues

All extra clues are important – for you will rarely get enough information from lip shape alone. Fortunately, you are not a beginner at making judgements from tone of voice, facial expression and so on. You have been doing it almost from the day you were born. You will be able to use this skill fully when lipreading.

Golden rules for you

Lipreading can never be as good as hearing – even if you are a star pupil.

Lipreading will flounder if the lighting is subdued or if people are moving about. Also if you are expected to do other things at the same time, like looking at photographs.

There are some golden rules to make things much easier for you and for those you want to hear.

Tell people you are deaf

Deafness does not show. Your ears look the same as anyone else's.

If you do not tell, the only way anyone can know is when you fail to understand. Then, more than likely, you will give the impression of being slow or tactless. It is better to tell at the outset, before you have something else to feel embarrassed about.

It should be easy, but it isn't. People like to feel good about themselves and it seems a poor start to a relationship to have to introduce yourself as someone who is below average in one particular respect. But do remember – it is only in one respect. Having a lousy pair of ears does not make you an inferior person.

Bluffing through may be possible for a short while – say for small talk with someone you meet while walking the dog. But if you want to talk for any length of time, the sooner you tell, the easier and less embarrassing it will be.

A lady was invited out to dinner by a man she had been eyeing for some weeks. She did not tell him she was deaf; and he wondered why she spent the whole evening leaning sideways. It was because the candles on the table were so tall that she could not see his mouth to lipread. The dim lighting did not help either. The evening was not a success.

Tell people how they can help

It's not a lot of use people knowing you are deaf if they don't know what to do about it.

They may shout, thinking that is enough – and then feel affronted when you are not grateful. Before that happens, you could make some suggestions that might help there and then:

Could I stand on the other side of you? This ear is better.

Most people will be only too happy to oblige.

Tell people if you have not understood

When you miss something in conversation, it may be tempting to keep quiet and hope it will come clear later. It might; but it might get worse. It will save a lot of time if you ask for repetition as soon as you feel at a loss, rather than wait until you have no idea what everyone is talking about.

Following a conversation under strain is exhausting. You may decide to bow out gracefully by simply not listening for a while – and just risk someone suddenly asking you a question. That is one option. But it is difficult to pick up the thread later or to judge when the topic has changed sufficiently to give you a fresh start.

If you have had enough, then retreat if you can. Start studying the pictures on the wall or leaf through a book. Go to the cloakroom or out for a short walk. Return to the group when you are ready. No-one will expect you to have heard anything in the meantime and so you can begin anew.

Golden rules for those who want to be heard

Make sure your face can be seen

For lipreading, the face and especially the mouth need to be clearly visible.

It is surprising how often something gets in the way. Tall house plants on the table, for example, make things difficult. So do newspapers – people have a tendency to read bits out from behind them.

People often move around when they are talking. If they are busy, cooking perhaps or making something, they open cupboards or look into tool bags as they speak. Then lipreading has to stop. If the person with you is hard of hearing, it is best to stop talking when you have to look elsewhere, and start again when you can be face to face.

Be face to face

Lipreading is easiest face to face. That does not mean you have to stand toe to toe. You can be at any angle so long as you can turn your head comfortably to face the person.

Most deaf people hear better with one ear than with the other. It is preferable to be on the side nearer to the better ear. This avoids the deaf person having to tilt his or her head to bring the better ear closer.

Be on the same level

It is better for both to be on the same level, either sitting or standing.

The distance between you should not be so short as to make it difficult for the deaf person to get an overall view of your face. It is not just the mouth he wants to see. He also gets clues from your facial expression and gestures

If he is too far away, he will be less able to use what hearing he does have. If it is noisy, he will need to get nearer to make hearing easier – but not too close that he cannot see what you are saying.

Noisy surroundings are a bad obstacle to hearing. Deaf people may turn off their hearing aids when the amplified noise becomes painful. Then they tend to move closer to get the best chance of hearing your voice.

There is no perfect solution. It makes sense to let a hard of hearing person choose the correct distance for the particular circumstances. This will probably be between three and six feet when it is reasonably quiet.

Avoid background noise

It is best to cut out background noise as much as you can. If possible, turn it off. If not, move to the least noisy part of the room.

The deaf usually prefer to sit in a corner, so that noise is not coming from all directions. Some say this sets up echoes and so prefer to be away from the wall. There are even some who are helped by noise and want to be near to it. As there is no hard and fast rule, let the deaf person choose.

Be in the light

Trying to lipread in subdued lighting, or with strobe lights, can be a nightmare. If you can control the lighting, make it bright and constant. Also make sure your face is not in shadow.

In daylight, it is usually best when the deaf person's back is to the window, so that light falls on the other's face. But the noise of traffic rumbling past, for example, may interfere with hearing.

The individual will know what is best at the time and should be allowed to choose.

Avoid echo chambers

A room with soft furnishings, carpet and curtains, will absorb unwanted noise and provide a good setting for conversation with a person who is hard of hearing.

Hard surfaces create echoes as the sound waves bounce off them. Too many, as in a workshop, tend to make speech unintelligible. So you may find someone who hears nothing when you are in the garage, with the engine running and your head under the bonnet, but has no difficulty at all when you go into the sitting room.

Get their attention first

Finally, just before you speak, make sure you have their attention.

The sound of a voice is enough to make hearing people turn towards the speaker. The deaf may not even hear the sound of the voice if they happen to be looking elsewhere.

Even if they do, they will not necessarily know who has spoken if there is more than one person in the room. There is a problem pinpointing where sound has come from. It is not even easy to judge whether the voice is male or female. So when deaf people hear a voice, they have to look from person to person to see whose mouth is moving. By that time, quite likely, someone else is talking. This can take several seconds to sort out and cause people to become flustered.

When it is discovered who is talking, the next task is to decipher the words. The bit missed may be vital – "It isn't true that... ". Working things out takes time and energy. Meanwhile people carry on talking.

This is another reason why the deaf sometimes give the impression of being simple. It is not that they could not understand as well as anyone else. But having missed vital bits of the speech, they are obliged to manage with less information – so they actually have to be cleverer just to seem normal.

To give the deaf a fair chance, attract their attention before you speak. Wave a hand, tap an arm or call them by name – clearly and fairly loudly, but without shouting. Pause for a moment to give them time to tune in. Start with something that does not need to be fully heard, like "Did you know?" or "By the way".

They will be far more likely to hear you clearly if you first do what you can do to make the conditions favourable.

Make the topic clear

People who hear easily will realise what the topic is in the first few words. They usually know at once if the subject is changed abruptly. Not so with the hard of hearing.

At first, the subject matter might be anything. If the deaf know what it is in advance, the words will be so much easier to work out.

For example, the words "jeep", "sheep" and "cheap" make similar mouth shapes. Knowing whether the topic is transport, farming or bargain hunting will make it easier to know which word is being used. No time need be wasted wondering why a dog is essential for the jeep.

Of course, there may be a farmer who wants a cheap jeep to transport sheep. Clear speech is essential.

Speak clearly

Clear speech means speaking so that it is easy to understand. It does not mean opening your mouth wide like a goldfish to express every syllable. That would make life impossible for a lipreader, for the lips are not forming a natural pattern. If you speak clearly, your lips will automatically form the right shape.

Your mouth will barely move if you mumble, so there will be little lip shape to go on. One lip shape will blur into the next if you gabble, and it will be difficult to sort out one from another.

Speaking clearly does not mean taking elocution lessons. It is like the difference between scribbling down a shopping list that only you will ever read, and writing a note for someone you do not know well. It means taking a bit more care.

Slow down a little bit

Some people, assuming the deaf to be brainless, talk... very... slowly... indeed. That is not necessary or helpful.

Those who don't hear easily do need extra time to work out a word and its meaning – but that time is measured in fractions of a second. It is helpful to slow down just a little and to pause slightly at the end of each sentence. But it is irritating to have everything drawn out forever.

It actually impedes understanding when words are spoken one at a time, with a gap between each. Neither the hearing nor the deaf can process information like that easily.

Information is divided into meaningful chunks with little words like "the" and "that" as fillers. We can manage without them, as we do in telegrams and headlines; and they certainly do not need to be emphasised.

I'm... going... to... the... shops... now.

Said like that, it is so long before the important word "shops" is uttered that the rest is forgotten. "What about the shops?", they ask. So the sentence is repeated even slower. This is asking for too much concentration for too long. Try talking like that to people who hear well. They too will find it hard to follow.

Instead, emphasise the important words that actually convey what is going to happen. I'm GOING to the SHOPS now.

The gap between "going" and "shops" is probably about right for the message to be easily understood. Also, talking like this is not so very far removed from normal speech. The deaf person will feel less like a village idiot.

Speak up a little bit

Speaking up means raising the volume just that little bit in order to make your voice clearer. It does not mean shouting. Damaged ears are less able to tolerate loud noise than ears in prime condition. You will probably get a wince in response if you shout. The ears hurt – but the sounds remain jumbled.

Keep your mouth clear

People move their hands about a lot. They stroke their chins, rub their noses and place fingers over their mouths. Some also move their heads about, flick their hair, and so on.

This is highly distracting to those who have to study the mouth as they listen. Try to hold your head reasonably still; and do keep your hands away from your mouth.

When it does not work

Try not to feel irritated if you have done all you can and the person still does not hear. Remember, it is more upsetting for the deaf than for you. They have to live with it all the time.

Don't make it into a big issue. Look straight at them, make sure there is nothing in front of your mouth and try again – perhaps a little louder and slower. If that doesn't work, try a different word or phrase. It could be that the words you used are especially difficult to lipread.

Gestures can help sometimes. When talking about swimming, you can make swimming movements with your arms. Don't overdo this for it can be distracting; and a mime that is obvious to you may seem obscure to someone else.

If that does not work, it saves time and embarrassment to write down the missing words. Please don't say "Never mind, it doesn't matter", even if it is trivial. The deaf person cannot help wondering what it was, and feel left out. There are too many different ways of getting the message across to make giving up acceptable.

Other methods of communicating

Most deaf people used speech for decades before it became difficult for them. That makes speech very much the preferred method of communication – but there are other ways. Most of these are used alongside speech. They add to it, rather than replace it.

Writing

Writing is an obvious way to help. It is quick and easy if pen and paper are at hand, and the skills needed are already in place. But a hunt for pen and paper may involve a lengthy wait. Nor is it always easy to stop and write things down – especially not outside in the rain, or in a moving queue for example.

Finger spelling

The finger spelling alphabet uses distinct finger patterns for each letter (see pages 50/51). Providing the conversing people both know it, a missed word can quickly be filled in by spelling it out with the fingers.

It is not sufficiently widely known to be relied on. Blue Peter, the children's programme, once tried to persuade the nation to learn it – but with only small success.

Finger spelling does not take long to learn. Most of the letters involve making the fingers look something like the letter itself. Children tend to master it in a few minutes. Adults take longer – but it is not a major undertaking.

With finger spelling, you have a quick and simple tool to make chit chat easy – that is if you can persuade your spouse, children and a few friends to learn it.

Cued speech

Cued speech is a way of using hand shapes (cues) to convey sounds, not letters. So the word "shop" starts with the hand shape for "sh", not with "s" as in finger spelling. It is used alongside speech and can be just as fast.

Cued speech is used to great effect with severely or profoundly deaf children who are at the stage of learning to speak. It is important for children to learn language early on, for it becomes far more difficult when delayed.

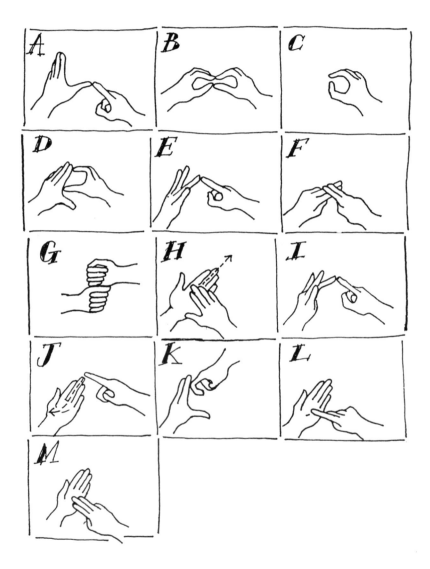

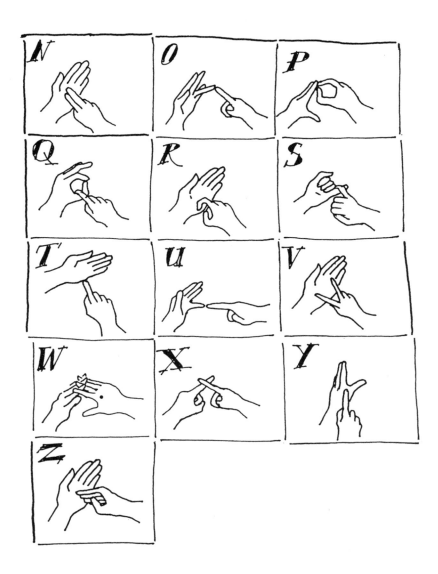

In cued speech, the cues are given at the same time as the words are spoken – so cues and lip shapes are learned together. It can also be used to help older children to catch up.

Some adults feel that cued speech is the answer to their problem. It can either be used continuously, or just now and then when lipreading fails. The cues are designed to clear up confusions of lip shapes. Those sounds that look similar on the lips, like "p", "b", and "m", are impossible to confuse in cued speech. That makes it useful as a prop to lipreading, especially when the words being said are difficult to lipread. It takes just a few hours to learn cued speech to this standard.

Cued speech conveys the identical message as the spoken word when it is known very well; and the deaf are no longer at a disadvantage.

Trained interpreters, called transliterators, enable the deaf to understand every word that is being said. This puts them on an equal footing with the hearing. Cued speech has been used successfully in law courts, hospitals and churches – all places where language needs to be understood precisely.

The National Centre for Cued Speech (see address list) runs courses for anyone who may be interested.

Sign language

Sign language is not often taken seriously by people who go deaf as adults. They tend to think either that it is not a proper language, or that it is too hard to learn. Neither assumption is true.

There are around 50,000 people in Britain who use sign language all the time. They converse freely on every topic under the sun, just like people who speak English.

Each country has its own sign language. In Britain it is British Sign Language (BSL). There is also Sign Supported English (SSE) which is much easier to learn.

In SSE there is a sign for every word, except for little words like "is", "the" and "of", which are left out (see examples on opposite page). "What's your name?" would involve using the signs for "What" then "your" then "name" – each sign accompanied by the spoken word.

BSL is different. Some signs correspond to English words and others do not. Nor is the order of the signs necessarily the same as the order of the words in English. "What's your name?" is signed "name, you?".

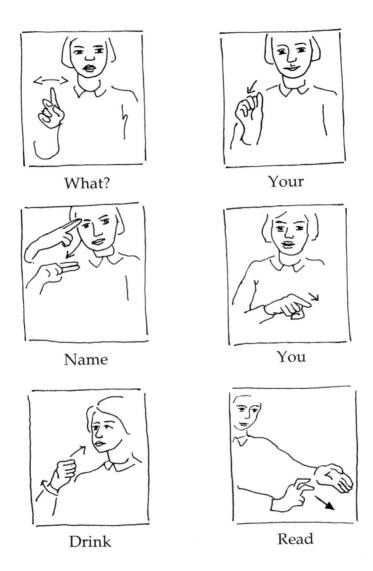

What?

Your

Name

You

Drink

Read

Some sentences are not remotely like English. "I was embarrassed because everybody was looking at me" is expressed in one sweeping movement. People using BSL do not speak at the same time – it wouldn't make sense.

Learning to use BSL fluently is a long-term project for which few people find enough time. Evening classes usually concentrate on SSE, with some BSL thrown in. This is something that can be picked up reasonably quickly.

Even knowing a dozen signs might make communication easier. For example, it was mentioned earlier that "to read" and "to drink" look similar on the lips. They do not look similar when signed. "Drink" is signed with a fist shape, tipped up towards the mouth like a drink. "Read" is signed by holding one hand out slightly bent, as though it were a book, and holding out the first two fingers of the other hand to represent eyes looking at the book and moving along it.

There are a lot of signs like that – obvious when you know what they mean. That makes them easy to learn. Some treat it as a kind of parlour game and go to sign language classes for fun. They are fun. Sign language classes are rocked with laughter.

If you like it and keep going, you will probably learn a few hundred signs. You may think that is of little use, as you know no-one else who knows sign language. The more people who say that, the fewer will bother to learn it and the less useful it will be.

Classes are becoming more popular. As time goes on, there should be more and more people who can sign. You can teach your family what you learn – and there are always your classmates. You will meet new people, get more support, talk more about hearing impairment and learn more ideas about what you can do.

Chapter 4
Hearing Aids

We know that people have been making hearing aids at least since the beginning of recorded history.

The first were made from natural objects like seashells and animal horns. They worked on the same principle as ear trumpets, by channelling soundwaves directly into the ear.

Ear trumpets work quite well; and more modern versions are still available for those whose fingers cannot manage fiddly controls or who cannot use a standard hearing aid because of some other handicap. There are people who simply prefer ear trumpets to modern hearing aids; and antique dealers are sometimes asked to seek them out.

The problem is that ear trumpets are conspicuous. That should not matter and, ideally, an ear trumpet should arouse no more comment than a pair of glasses or a walking stick – but it does! Those embarrassed about hearing loss want to conceal it for as long as possible; and a long tube sticking out of the side of their heads is certainly not acceptable.

People went to great lengths to hide ear trumpets when they were the only available form of hearing aid. Some were built into hats, fans and walking sticks and hidden that way. The most ingenious camouflage was a throne, specially commissioned by King Jaõ V1 of Portugal in 1819. It had two long tubes that went from ear height down to the arm rests, which were ornately decorated with the heads of roaring lions. The king's subjects spoke into the lions' mouths and the soundwaves moved up the tubes to the royal ears. It was, despite the frills, basically just another ear trumpet.

The first electrical aids were made around the beginning of this century; but those were very cumbersome. By the late 1940s, transistors had enabled more manageable versions to be produced. Since then, the electronic boom has made smaller and smaller models possible.

Types of hearing aid

Behind-the-ear

This is the most common type available.

An earmould, which has to be a precise fit, is placed in the ear. This is connected by a flexible tube to the actual hearing aid (consisting of microphone, battery and controls) which is contained in a plastic box behind the ear.

In-the-ear

In this type, the electronics are all housed within the earmould in the ear.

There is nothing needed behind the ear; and consequently there is far less to see than with a behind-the-ear aid. But the aid is still clearly visible to anyone who bothers to look.

In-the-ear-canal

Some models – smaller and less noticeable – fit right inside the ear canal; but the controls are also smaller and require nimble fingers to operate. Also, this type of aid requires more cleaning than other models as it is sited close to the glands that produce wax.

Body-worn aids

Body-worn aids are pocket-sized units attached to an earmould in the ear via a cord. The units are clipped on to clothing or worn in a pouch around the neck.

These are more powerful and have easier controls to manage than those within the ear.

Problems may sometimes be caused by clothes moving and rubbing around the aid. The sounds caused by this movement are picked up by the hearing aid and can be so amplified as to become troublesome and even to blot out speech altogether.

Bone-conduction aids

Bone-conduction aids are most suitable for those with middle ear damage. They bypass the middle ear altogether and, using the bone behind the ear, conduct sound straight to the inner ear.

This type of aid does not require an earmould. It is very useful therefore where ears are prone to infection or are inclined to become watery.

There are some disadvantages though. It takes a lot of amplification to get sound through the bone, so the batteries are quickly used up. Also, it is difficult to get just the right amount of pressure on the bone – hard enough to conduct sound properly but not so hard as to be uncomfortable.

Bone-anchored hearing aid (BAHA)

This new type of aid also works by conduction of sound through bone. In this case, the aid is attached to a kind of press stud screwed into the skull.

A special screw, which will not rust or rot, is inserted in a hole drilled into the bone of the skull. It then takes about three months for the bone to grow tight around the screw, which can then be used as an anchorage point for the new aid.

At the time of writing (late 1993), this type of aid has already been tried on 450 patients in 21 hospitals. If all goes well, it is hoped to increase its rate of use to 500 patients a week.

Spectacle aids

Hearing aids can be incorporated into glasses.

The components are contained within the arm of the spectacles and attached to an earmould in the ear (or to a vibrator behind the ear in the case of bone conduction).

If you need both glasses and a hearing aid, it is simpler to have one piece of equipment rather than two. But if either one needs changing, it is more complicated than if they were separate.

CROS

CROS stands for "Co-lateral routing of signals". To make it easier to remember, think that it makes the sound CROS(S) from one ear to the other.

This is a useful type of aid for those who have one bad ear and one good. There is a microphone in the bad ear and a receiver in the good one.

This can work well in situations like meetings, where it is necessary to hear people from more than one direction. Also in the car, if the good ear is on the side farther away from the other person.

CROS aids are generally incorporated into glasses.

BICROS

BICROS aids exist for those who have two bad ears – but with one ear better than the other.

In this case, a microphone in each ear mixes the sound and sends it to a receiver sited in the better ear.

Special features of some hearing aids

Peak clipping

Noise is clipped when it reaches a certain peak level.

This helps with loudness discomfort by not allowing noise to reach a level at which it hurts.

Tone control

Hearing loss almost always first affects high frequencies. So low frequencies, like deep voices, may be heard quite well even when high voices are not. Sometimes it is the other way round.

A hearing aid with tone control can be set so that some frequencies are amplified in preference to others. This can help the problem of background noise (mostly of low frequency) if the control is set so as not to amplify the low frequencies.

Automatic gain control

The amplifier automatically turns itself down as the noise gets louder.

This makes the volume of sound heard more even and reduces the need to fiddle constantly with the volume control, which is one of the bugbears of using a hearing aid.

Automatic push-pull circuitry

This is a power saving device that helps to cut down battery use.

Getting the hearing aid

The NHS provides hearing aids free on permanent loan. Batteries and maintenance are also provided free. Aids can also be bought from private dispensers. The pros and cons of each method of supply are discussed later in this chapter.

Whoever provides it, that part of the hearing aid that goes inside your ear (the earmould) must be made specially for you. It has to be a snug fit, for any air gaps will create an effect called "acoustic feedback" – a high-pitched whistle delivered straight into your ear. Looking around at ears will convince you of the amazing variety of their shapes and sizes. The only way to get a snug fit therefore is to have a cast taken of your ear.

Making the cast

A white substance is squirted into your ear. It may feel cold but it is not painful in any way. It hardens after a minute or so and can be taken out.

There then follows a wait of some weeks until the earmould is made and the hearing aid fitted. The length of time involved varies from clinic to clinic.

Fitting the hearing aid

You are not likely to forget your first day with a hearing aid. It is not at all easy to get used to wearing one; and it can even seem hopeless at times. You just have to keep on telling yourself that this strange object is an electronic marvel that will, given the chance, help greatly in your everyday life.

The hearing aid most usually tried first is the NHS behind-the-ear type. The following description applies to that type. Others may be easier or more difficult to fit but the basic problems remain the same.

First you will be shown the aid and told how it works and how to insert the batteries. The controls usually consist of a volume control knob and another switch with three positions. These are M (for microphone, meaning "on"), T (for telecoil, for use with loop systems as explained in chapters 5 and 6), and O (for off).

You will be shown how to put the earmould into your ear. This is when you first realise that you have never seen the inside of your ear and have no idea what it looks like. You still will not be able to see it; and inserting the mould is like trying to do a three dimensional jigsaw with your eyes shut. You push and heave and hope – while the expert watches.

It fits easily enough, once you get the knack. It is a matter of inserting it at the right angle and turning it by the right amount. Make sure that the top bit of the earmould is in the ridge at the top of your ear – it was designed to fit in there.

The main unit of the aid is then dangling down. You have to place it behind your ear without twisting the tube that links the aid to the ear-mould. Remember that sound has to travel through that tube; and that you will hear nothing if it is twisted. You can tell whether or not it is twisted by feeling along it with your finger and thumb. If it is twisted, then try again.

You can try out the aid once it is in place. By now though, you will probably have forgotten about the controls. You can't see them – so you have to feel around.

What to expect

Don't expect normal hearing to occur as soon as you find the switch. You may just get whistling. That probably means you did not get the earmould in right. Push it around a bit more and try again.

Another possibility is that you get a continuous buzz. That means that the switch has been set to "T" when there is no loop system. Have another stab at the switch.

You may, of course, get nothing at all. That could be because you have turned off the appliance, or else turned the volume control to zero when you were feeling around.

Keep fiddling about. Eventually, you will get a sound resembling speech – assuming the person with you is talking at the moment you get it right.

Don't worry about it sounding odd. Voices heard through a hearing aid have a mechanical quality about them that takes some getting used to. You will become accustomed to it in time.

Learning to use a hearing aid

It is not known how many hearing aids have been stuffed into the back of a drawer and forgotten – but the number must be huge. Most hearing aids are a disappointment at first. It is not that they cannot help, given time; but that people expect too much of them and far too soon.

After not hearing properly for some time, it comes as a shock to hear all sounds amplified. Suddenly you are able to hear footsteps, the sound of typewriters clacking and of kettles whistling. All this noise interferes with the sound (like speech) you really want to hear. You have to learn to block out all the extra noise, while tuning in to the people talking to you – and that takes a lot of practice.

It may sometimes be harder, with a hearing aid, to hear someone talking than without one – so you may switch it off. You then find that the earmould has become an effective ear plug, making matters worse than ever. So what's the point? The temptation to stuff the hearing aid into a drawer is strong.

Many try too hard. Having gone to the trouble of getting a hearing aid, they want to use it all the time and expect an immediate and dramatic result. But a hearing aid is not a magic wand. It is a tool designed to help you re-learn the skill of hearing.

With most skills, people accept that they must start with the easy bits and work up gradually. That is also what you need to do with a hearing aid.

Make everything as easy as you can at first. Extra noises make it more difficult, so choose a quiet room. It is harder when you are tired, so make it early in the day. It is easier with familiar voices, so be with people you know – but only with one person at a time at first. It is not an endurance test, so don't go at it for too long. Put the hearing aid away when using it becomes a strain. More practice later.

Do not start using the aid in more difficult situations until you have become accustomed to it. Try it first with two or three people in a quiet place, then at a dinner table where the noise of crockery and cutlery can be distracting. Later, you could start taking it out with you; but put it away if it gets too noisy.

Going at your own pace, you should gradually increase the amount you use the hearing aid. You will never have to take an exam in its use. How much you eventually use it is entirely up to you.

Go back to whoever supplied the hearing aid if, after a trial period, you decide that it does not help you. You may be able to try another type that suits you better.

Fine, if you decide in the end that hearing aids are not for you. But do give them a fair trial. They are often disappointing at first but prove to be a boon in the end.

Care of your hearing aid

Cleaning

The earmould should be cleaned at least once a week. This is to get rid of any accumulated wax which, though not harmful, will block off the sound.

Do remember always that the electronic components must never get wet.

With a behind-the-ear aid, carefully pull the tubing away from the main unit. Do this by holding the hard plastic tube close to the body of the aid in one hand, and gently pulling out the flexible tubing with the other.

Don't pull the tubing out of the earmould except when you have to replace it. Wash the earmould, together with the flexible tube attached to it, in warm soapy water. Then rinse thoroughly and dry with a towel or soft cloth. Blowing down the tube, and gently tapping the earmould at the same time, helps to dislodge any water droplets stuck inside. Finally, place the earmould in a warm place for an hour or so to get rid of condensation.

Make sure the tube is facing the right way when you re-attach it to the main unit of the hearing aid. The side with the smooth curve goes towards the unit behind the ear. Put the earmould in your ear if you are unsure and keep your thumb on the back when you take it out. Then push the tubing back onto the hard plastic tube attached to the main unit.

For body-worn aids, pull the earmould away from the receiver and wash the earmould as for a behind-the-ear aid. Take advice from the supplier for all in-the-ear and in-the-ear-canal aids. The electrical components are inside the earmould and must not get wet. Special wax-removing agents are available for use.

Batteries

Batteries can last for anything from three days to several weeks, depending on the type and how often they are used.

Body-worn aids require penlight batteries, which are inserted in the same way as in a torch. You will get a warning that they are running low when the sound level starts to fade.

Other hearing aids use coin-shaped batteries. You need always to carry at least one spare with you – for this type of battery suddenly stops working without warning when exhausted.

The supplier will show you how to insert the battery. It can be difficult to see which way up it goes. There is a + sign on the battery which should be matched with the + sign marked on the aid. But you do need good eyesight. If the hearing aid does not work after putting in a new battery, try it the other way up. Some hearing aids make it easier by making it impossible to close the lid of the battery compartment when the battery is upside-down.

The NHS initially provides you with two packs of six batteries. When one pack is used, you return it in exchange for a new set – so you always have one packet in use and one in reserve. One way of distinguishing dead batteries from live ones is to put them back in the container upside down.

You are expected to return the dead batteries, which are promptly replaced by new ones. In some areas you can do this by post. It is vital to keep batteries out of reach if you have children or animals in your house, for they are small and easily swallowed.

Get medical attention immediately if this happens or if you think it may possibly have happened.

Re-tubing the earmould

Behind-the-ear aids come with a flexible tube connecting the earmould and the main body of the aid. This tube hardens in time. It may crack after a few months and have to be replaced. In some cases the tubing is cemented into place and so can only be replaced by the supplier. But mostly this is a job you can do yourself.

Sometimes, the tubing is attached to a rigid elbow at both ends. Then you simply pull each end away, cut another piece of tubing to the same length as the old one, and push the new one back into place.

In many cases, there is just a rigid elbow at the aid end and the other end is threaded through the earmould. This type is trickier but not too difficult to replace.

The supplier probably showed you how to do it on the day the hearing aid was first fitted – but you had a lot to think about then and have probably forgotten. There is no need to feel foolish as you struggle to remember. Like many things, it is easy when you know how – and nearly impossible when you do not.

You do need supple fingers. If that is a problem, or for any reason you find you cannot do it, the supplier will do it for you – free if it is an NHS aid and sometimes free with a private one. That means taking it to the supplier's premises, or posting it and managing without the aid until the postman returns it to you. It is more convenient to do it yourself if you can. Here's how …

1   *Remove the old tube by tugging it free.*

2   *Cut a length of new tubing about an inch-and-a-half longer than the old.*

3   *The new tube needs a pointed end in order to thread it through the ear-mould. So prepare a sharp point by making a diagonal cut at the end, and then a second diagonal cut in the other direction.*

4   *The tubing has to go from the outside of the earmould to the inside. If you are in doubt as to which is the outside, put the earmould in your ear and keep a finger on the outside as you take it out again.*
    Poke the pointed end of the tube into the hole and push it through. Keep on pushing until the point is sticking out at the other end.

5   *Cut off the point. Then file down the end of the tubing until none protrudes from the hole. A hard edge of plastic would feel uncomfortable if pressed against your ear.*

6   *There is now a length of new tubing coming from the outside of the ear-mould. Stick the other end of this tube into the rigid elbow attached to the aid.*

7   *Put the hearing aid on. You have done it!*

Changing the cord

On body-worn aids, there is a cord between the receiver and the amplifier. This can become brittle and may need replacing after a few months.

This is a simple job. You just unplug the old and plug in the new.

Looking after your hearing aid

Remember to switch off your hearing aid before you take it out. It will whistle if you forget – but you may not hear it and other members of the family may spend time tracking down the funny noise. If nobody notices, you are likely to have a dead battery before long.

Keep the hearing aid dry. It will not survive if you wash your hair when wearing it. Keep it away from hair-care preparations altogether. Hair spray (and other sorts of spray) may clog up the works or even melt the plastic.

There is a chance that the batteries may explode if they get too hot. So keep the aid away from the hair dryer. Remove the battery if you do not expect to wear the aid for some time. Otherwise it may corrode and damage the appliance. Keep your hearing aid away from the dog. The NHS takes a dim view of replacing chewed-up hearing aids and you may be asked to pay for a new one.

Problem checklist

Like most other devices, hearing aids can go wrong. Any fault in the electrical components will need a professional repairer. In that case, take it back to the supplier. There will be no charge if it is an NHS aid. It is inconvenient though, so first check that it is not a simple job you can do yourself.

Little or no sound

- Check the volume control. The setting may not be high enough.
- Check the tubing. This may be twisted.
  If not, it may be blocked by condensation – then it will usually be misted over. Pull the tubing free of the rigid elbow at the aid end. Keeping it attached to the earmould, blow sharply down it to dislodge the moisture. Tapping the earmould gently at the same time may help. If necessary, leave it in a warm place for a while to dry out thoroughly.
- Check the battery. This may be the wrong way up.
  With a body-worn aid, try cleaning the contacts and connections. If none of that helps, try a new battery.
- Check the cord. For a body-worn aid, try replacing it.
- Check the earmould. This may be blocked with wax.
  Wash it in warm soapy water and rinse well, remembering that any trace of soap can block the sound. Leave it in a warm place until thoroughly dry.

Extra noises

- Buzzing. This probably means the switch is on "T" when there is no loop system.
- Whistling. This is usually the result of air getting in somewhere. Check that the earmould fits snugly in your ear. If it still whistles, check the tubing which may have split. Replace it if necessary. If it still whistles, you may have excess wax in your ear. Go to your GP.

- Crackling sound. There is probably a faulty connection somewhere. On a body-worn aid, you can try replacing the cord, or just cleaning it or cleaning the volume control. If that does not help, return the aid to the supplier for repair.

  With behind-the-ear and smaller aids, this is a job for the professional.

NHS or private?

The NHS provides a comprehensive service, supplying, fitting, and maintaining hearing aids free of charge. The private sector does the same – but with much more choice – for a charge.

Procedure

After first telling a doctor that you are concerned about your hearing, you will go through the same procedures whether you use the NHS or private health care.

Once it has been decided that you need a hearing aid, the choice of aid is no longer just a medical matter. A hearing aid will neither improve nor detract from the condition of your ears. It is merely an attempt to alleviate the symptoms of a condition that is not amenable to treatment or cure.

Fitting

The fitting of hearing aids is a skilled job that requires thorough training. The person who fits the aid will necessarily have detailed knowledge of the ear and how it works in normal circumstances, as well as being aware of what might go wrong.

He or she may also be a doctor; but full medical qualifications are not required at this stage. You will be advised if you should have medical treatment rather than a hearing aid.

You can go right through the process, from the first consultation to fitting the hearing aid, on the NHS or privately. You can even swop midstream from one system to the other if you wish. It is entirely up to you.

Choice

The main difference is that of choice. The NHS has a restricted range of aids and will issue the same type to thousands of people.

The private sector can provide every possible type, with each aid adjusted to the needs of the individual user. The latest technological advances usually become available in the private sector long before they filter through to the NHS.

It could be that the NHS aid suits your needs very well. In that case you would end up with a similar product from a private dispenser. Since hearing aids cost hundreds of pounds, it makes sense to try the free version first. Even if you find it hopeless, it will give you some experience in using one. You will then know what questions to ask if you eventually decide to go private.

Dispensers

You may still hear occasional horror stories about cowboy salesmen – but these date from long ago and have probably been much exaggerated in the telling. Consumer protection laws have done much to root out such practices. The standard advice is to stick to established firms of good reputation – but that is hard on anyone trying to start up.

Every hearing aid dispenser must, by law, be registered with the Hearing Aid Council and must abide by its Code of Practice. The person who sees you will either be a fully qualified hearing aid dispenser, or a trainee under supervision. The customer must be told if a hearing aid is not likely to help, and be directed to a doctor if it is thought that the deafness may be treatable.

Comparison of services

Waiting

A private dispenser will see you in a matter of days.

The NHS could take months, depending on the waiting list in your area. Your local hospital may be one of the quicker ones, so do enquire.

Home visits

Private dispensers are more than willing to visit you in your own home – even if you are able-bodied and live in a remote area. This has the important advantage that you can see how the aid performs in situations you find difficult – like when the tap is running or the television is on.

A consulting room, which provides the almost ideal hearing conditions of one to one in a quiet room, can give you a false impression of how good the aid is.

Some people are reluctant to let salesmen into their homes for fear they will not get them out again without signing on the dotted line. If you do sign on your own premises without meaning to, or change your mind later, the law provides a cooling-off period during which you can cancel without losing any money.

Some dispensers automatically visit everyone who makes an enquiry. So be sure to make it clear if you do not want a home visit.

Tests

NHS tests are free. Some private tests are also free. Some private dispensers charge a fee but refund it if you buy an aid from them.

Both ears should be tested – even if one seems reasonable and you only want one aid. It is sometimes recommended that the aid goes in the better ear!

The usual hearing test uses pure tones – a series of bleeps of high, medium and low pitch. This is a good way of measuring hearing loss. But you need more help with speech than just with bleeping noises, so you should ask for a speech discrimination test as well.

Fitting

The fitting should not be hurried. People need guidance and reassurance at this time.

A "Which?" report (August 1993) found that private customers get more time. They are given over half an hour in most cases, whereas most NHS patients get less than 20 minutes.

Advice

The same "Which?" report found that NHS customers got fuller advice even though their time was shorter. NHS staff gave extra information about other devices, like special alarm clocks, support services and lipreading classes. They were also more likely to refer the patient on to other agencies, like social services, who can supply equipment free of charge.

Types of aid available

At present, the NHS mainly provides behind-the-ear and body-worn aids. It plans to start supplying in-the-ear ones as well, but not necessarily all over the country. This will be the decision of each local health authority.

Private dispensers provide every type of aid and will continue to add new types as technology progresses. This is a particular advantage if the private dispenser runs a rental scheme – for you will then be able to update your model quickly.

The development work described in Chapter 8 of this book will eventually result in vastly improved and more sensitive hearing aids; and it is more than likely that these will first become available in the private sector.

Free trial periods

Private dispensers are understandably reluctant to allow you to take away a device worth several hundred pounds without paying anything.

Most will ask you to pay a deposit, and then give you a period of up to thirty days during which you can bring it back for a full refund – for any reason!

Follow-up

You should get as many follow-up appointments as you need to iron out any problems.

Both the NHS and the private sector will provide these. The NHS makes no charge. The private sector may or may not, depending on the circumstances and what has been agreed.

Servicing

The NHS makes no charge for servicing or maintenance.

In the private sector, the price of the aid often also covers lifelong servicing. In that case, the only additional cost is for batteries.

Batteries

NHS batteries are free. You are also entitled to them if they are the right sort for your private aid.

Other types of battery are readily available from hearing aid dispensers and chemists. A penny buys about five hours of use. They have a long shelf life – so you can stock up.

NHS *and private – combined*

The NHS may pay for a private aid if you can convince them that your case is exceptional – but they take a lot of convincing! They might look more favourably on the idea if you find loud noises painful, or if you have lost most of your hearing very suddenly – like after an accident or an infection.

Another possibility is to have one NHS aid and one private one. Two hearing ears are better than one – for you get sound from all around, need not twist your head about and get a better idea of where the sound is coming from. The NHS may prescribe two aids – but this is unusual.

Prices

The "Which?" report mentioned earlier found that recommended retail prices ranged from £199 for a behind-the-ear aid, to £1,299 for a programmable one that will adapt to different situations. The most expensive behind-the-ear aid was only £4 less than this, at £1,295.

I obtained three quotes for aids to correct my own hearing loss – £275, £395 and £450, or double that for two. The aids recommended were similar but not identical. With the cheapest, there was a charge for the hearing test (refundable if I bought an aid) and a charge for servicing. The most expensive was the best. I got the same general advice from all three.

Deciding

This is rarely a straightforward decision and it depends very much on personal circumstances and priorities.

You need not hesitate if the NHS aid suit you. On the other hand, if a particular privately supplied aid can give you an additional degree of ease and comfort, this must be good value if you can afford it. For those who readily spend many thousands of pounds on a new car, the choice should be easy.

Don't buy in a hurry. Take it as a bad sign if you are pressurised, for a reputable salesman will not try to force you into a hasty decision. Just walk away. You can always come back, or go somewhere else, if you later decide you were getting good advice.

No hearing aid can restore normal hearing. Flee from any salesman who suggests that it can. Beware if words like "magic" or "miracle" are used.

Take someone with you for moral support if you are not very good at saying no.

You want the right features for the right price, and with the right terms and conditions. It pays to shop around – just as you would for a washing machine or a new car. Your hearing aid may well be a far more important purchase.

Chapter 5
More Technical Help

"Assistive devices" is the term used for devices, other than hearing aids, that can assist the hard of hearing.

There are different ones for different purposes. There are devices for use with the television, others for the telephone and yet others for public meetings. Wherever there is a need to hear, you will find some kind of device designed to help. Some are available free of charge from Social Services – it is worth asking.

Some devices just make the sound extra-loud, like special alarm clocks. Others use advanced technology to channel sound straight into earphones. A different kind gets rid of the need to hear at all; and uses lights or vibrating pads instead.

Alarm clocks

There is a wide choice of alarm clocks available. These look similar to ordinary clocks; and there is the same choice – digital or analogue, mains or battery operated, snooze control and bedside light. The difference lies in the additional features – extra volume, flashing lights and vibrating pads.

- Extra loud. If you want to use sound, some ordinary clocks may be loud enough – ask to hear them in the shop.
  There is one, designed for deaf children, that makes a noise like a cock crowing very loudly.
- Flashing lights. Instead of a bell ringing, a light flashes on and off at the appointed hour. These lights can also be used as bedside lights.
- Vibrating pads. A vibrating pad can be plugged into the clock. The pad goes under the pillow and vibrates at a pre-set time. Though any sound it makes will be muffled by the pillow, the vibrations are very effective at waking people up.

There is also a battery-operated alarm clock, designed to go under the pillow – the whole clock. It simply shakes you awake at getting-up time.

Doorbells

There is a wide range of doorbells, most of which have an ordinary bell in addition to their special features. Some can be installed by a competent amateur. Others need a qualified electrician.

- Extra loud. A transformer, mounted on the wall, makes the bell loud enough for quite a severe hearing loss.
- Lights. There is a unit for bedsits and small flats that can be plugged into the mains and has a lamp that doubles as a reading lamp. The only wiring required is between the bell and the unit.
  When the bell rings, the light also flashes. This can also be connected to the phone, so that the light flashes in time to the ringing.
  Larger systems use the normal lighting in the house. It is very startling when all the lights start flashing – especially at night. There is an option for use at night, when the lights are dimmed. Alternatively, special low-voltage lights (amber coloured) can be installed.
- Vibrators. This works in conjunction with a loop system, which is a means of directing sound direct to the user.
  A vibrator is carried in the pocket or clipped on to the clothes. When the bell rings, it sends a signal via the loop to the vibrator. It can work up to a range of 100 metres.
- Hearing aid connection. It is possible, with a loop system, to send the sound of the doorbell straight to the hearing aid.

Smoke detectors

Smoke detectors are increasingly being used as a basic precaution – and not just for the deaf. They can detect small amounts of smoke, and will sound (or flash or vibrate) a warning while it is still easy to breathe in comfort and escape. They are operated by battery and easy to install.

Smoke detectors make a loud noise; but if there is a risk of sleeping through it, optional extras, such as a vibrator or strobe lights or both, may also be added.

The control pack goes near the bed. It contains the batteries and usually has an indicator light to show that they are still working. The pack has two sockets – one for the vibrator and one for a strobe light. Either or both may be used.

The vibrator can go under the pillow or under the mattress. The strobe lights should be placed within sight of the bed. Either system on its own should wake even the deepest sleeper. To be safer than safe, you can use both.

The actual detector goes on or close to the ceiling adjacent to the bedroom. The smoke will first start collecting under the ceiling and will activate the alarm well before it has become thick enough to be dangerous.

Microphone pick up

This is a multi-purpose device that detects sound in one room and causes a light to flash in another.

It consists of two parts. The transmitter with microphone is placed near the sound source – doorbell, telephone, baby, etc. The portable receiver is taken into the room where the deaf person is, and plugged into the mains.

The microphone picks up the sound, which is transmitted by the existing house wiring to the portable receiver. A button-sized light on the receiver flashes in time to the sound. So if the baby whimpers, it will flash now and then. If the baby starts bawling, it will flash continuously.

More than one transmitter can be used; and then a different light will flash, depending on which room the sound is coming from. Some models can also be used in conjunction with a vibrator under the pillow.

Television

The following devices can also be used with audio systems and radios.

Listening aids

These consist of a microphone, a receiver unit and an earphone.

The microphone is put close to the speaker on the TV set and secured in place with a velcro sticker. The microphone plug goes into the receiver unit which delivers the sound direct to the earphone in the deaf person's ear.

There is a volume control on the receiver, separate from the one on the television, so that the user can have a louder volume than the rest of the family.

There is also a version that plugs straight into the jack socket (or into the mains isolator unit if there is no jack socket) to eliminate the need for a microphone.

These aids, with the exception of the loop system, mostly do not require the use of a hearing aid.

Loop system

The loop is a well-known system, often found in public buildings. It consists of a control box, a microphone and a long piece of wire.

On domestic systems, the wire is long enough to go round a large living room with some to spare. Both ends of the wire are plugged into the back of the control unit. This makes a large loop of wire, from which the system gets its name.

The loop is arranged around the room and concealed under the carpet or attached to the skirting. If there is wire left over, this must be coiled up and not cut, or the system won't work.

A microphone is plugged into the unit and attached to the television (close to its speaker) with the velcro tabs provided. Then the unit is plugged into the mains.

When it is switched on, sound is delivered straight to the hearing aid, which must be switched to "T". The loop is like a perimeter fence for hearing. So long as you are inside it, all the sound going through the microphone reaches your ear. Other sounds do not – so there is no distracting background noise. This makes the sound you want to hear much clearer. The loop works beautifully for many people.

A disadvantage is that other voices count as background noise and are cut out. You will not therefore hear the person sitting next to you unless that person is also wearing a microphone. Domestic loop systems are provided with two microphone sockets so that you can talk to one other person at the same time as you watch television.

In theory, you can move around and still hear the television – as long as you stay within the confines of the loop. But you will stop hearing as soon as you step outside it. It is not so clear cut in practice. There are "deaf spots" inside the loop; and you may lose the sound if you move around or even lean back. At the same time, it may work for you outside the loop – maybe several feet away. Some people can go to the kitchen and prepare a snack without missing any dialogue.

Infra-red systems

A transmitter is plugged in near the television and a microphone is attached to it, close to its speaker.

The sound is transmitted in the form of an infra-red signal all around the room. There are no wires between the television and the people listening. The user, or users, wear headphones.

This system can be used with any number of people. Each set of headphones has its own volume control. Some are fitted with an inductive coupler – which means it can be used with the "T" switch of a hearing aid if preferred – but the sound may be clear enough without a hearing aid at all.

Subtitles

You can have subtitles on some programmes with a teletext television. The number of programmes provided with subtitles is increasing all the time, and the television companies have promised more.

Most video recorders do not record the subtitles; but it is possible to buy or rent ones that do. Videos with subtitles can be hired from video rental firms and local libraries. The range is rather limited at the moment – but the more they are asked for, the sooner a better range will be provided.

VideoCaptions

There is a non-profit-making enterprise called the VideoCaption Service that aims to provide a steady flow of videos with closed captions.

The letters of these captions are in white and they are encased in a black box which makes them easy to read. To make it even easier, the subtitle moves about the screen to the person who is speaking.

Videos with these captions have labels marked with a symbol (see illustration page 80) that looks like a cross between a television screen and a speech bubble in a comic.

Some hearing people are irritated by subtitles and would not buy or hire a video using them – and this makes marketing difficult.

The VideoCaption Service solves that problem by giving the choice to the consumer. The subtitles do not actually appear unless a special device, called a VideoCaption Reader, is installed. You simply plug it in to the television and video. It is a portable device, only about the size of a video case, so you can take it with you when you go visiting. It is a useful piece of equipment for baby sitters whose charges sleep peacefully all evening.

VideoCaption Readers are obtainable from Blockbusters, Radio Rentals and Ritz stores. They can also be ordered from Sound Advantages (see address list). Their price (February 1994) is around £100 plus VAT. The registered deaf or hard of hearing are exempt from VAT; and your supplier will have a special form that exempts you from having to pay the VAT. That is a good reason to get yourself registered (see page 85).

Digital sound

Some televisions use a digital sound system. This is designed to improve the sound quality for everyone, and not just for the deaf. It might be helpful to you, depending on your particular hearing loss.

If you are thinking of buying a new television, ask to hear those with digital sound first. Many modern records, tapes and compact discs also use digital sound. It is worth a try.

Telephones

There are two problems with telephones – hearing them ring and then hearing what is said.

Starting with the simplest techniques, a phone will ring louder if it is on a hard surface rather than on the soft padding of a telephone table. You could put it in a biscuit tin to produce an echo effect.

Moving up the technological scale, many modern phones have a volume control knob. On some, the pitch can also be varied to suit your hearing loss.

There is other help to hand if you still cannot hear the telephone at maximum volume.

Extension bells

These are extra-loud bells fixed to the wall. There is also an outdoor version.

Extension tonecaller

This has a very loud ring which is adjustable by a volume control. It also has a tone control with a choice of four different tones.

Installation is easy if you have a modern phone socket. First pull the phone cord out of the socket. Push in a double socket plug (available from

BT). You then have two sockets. Put the tonecaller cord in one and the telephone cord in the other.

The tonecaller is attached to the wall by two screws and BT provide a template for you to position them. Alternatively, simply put it on a convenient shelf.

Tonecallers and extension bells can be provided free of charge to hearing-impaired residential customers. If you have had one for some time and are paying rental for it, call BT on 150 and they will stop charging you from the date of your call.

Flashing lights

Some telephones incorporate a light which flashes when the phone rings.

Microphone pick up

This has already been described above.

A microphone near the telephone activates a light in another room. A possible problem with this is that the light may flash in response to other noises, such as the dog barking. It usually flashes in synchrony with the noise – which helps. But there is a device that can be coupled with the telephone line and which responds only to the ringing of the phone. A vibrating pad can also be used.

A leaflet called Alerting Devices can be obtained by phoning the Royal National Institute for Deaf People (RNID) on 0800 413 114.

Speech amplifiers

Some phones come with a control that allows you to turn up the volume of the voice at the other end – or your own voice if you are speaking to someone with hearing difficulties – or both.

Some can also be adjusted to enhance high frequency sounds, which makes speech clearer for deaf people.

Inductive couplers

Some phones, including all public pay phones and motorway emergency phones, have inductive couplers for use with the "T" switch on the hearing aid.

If you have a body-worn aid, you will need to hold the phone upside down, so that the sound goes into the receiver of the aid.

Strap-on earpieces

You can buy a small battery-operated earpiece with an amplifier or inductive coupler or both. This straps on to the earpiece of your phone.

You will probably have to remove it when you finish the call as, with most phones, it prevents the handset from being properly replaced.

Extra earpieces

Some types of phone can be fitted with an additional earpiece, with or without an inductive coupler. This enables you to listen with both ears, which may help.

Alternatively, a hearing person can also listen in – and then relay the message to the deaf person. It is easier to understand someone sitting beside you than a disembodied voice.

If the phone is suitable, BT will supply this earpiece free of charge to hearing-impaired residential customers.

Textphones and minicoms

Textphones are for people who cannot hear a voice on the phone. There is a keyboard, like on a typewriter, and a screen at both ends. A minicom is a portable version of this.

The message is typed in. It appears on the screen of the phone being used and on the screen of the phone being called. More and more companies are having textphones installed. They have the word "text" or "minicom" next to their phone number in the directory.

Typetalk

This is a service set up to help minicom users to telephone people who have no minicom, and the other way round.

It is not possible to dial direct – so Typetalk becomes the middle man. An operator (who has signed a confidentiality contract) listens to the hearing person, types what is said to the deaf person, receives back the typed message and then speaks to the hearing person. Or if preferred, the deaf person can speak directly to the hearing person, and receive the reply typed.

The service is available at any time, day or night, throughout the year – and to most countries in the world.

Financial help

As it takes longer to type than to talk, textphone calls are more expensive than the equivalent spoken ones. This is recognised as being unfair, so steps have been taken to deal with this.

There is a text-users' rebate scheme, which entitles non-business customers to a 60% rebate on their phone bill – up to a maximum of £160 per year.

Typetalk is even more expensive, as every word has to be relayed twice – once by voice and once by text. There is a scheme, involving a lot of arithmetic, to reduce the cost to what it would have been if both parties could hear.

Directory enquiries

Directory enquiries now use electronic voices, which can pose a problem for the hard of hearing. If that applies to you, tell the operator, who will see to it that you get a human voice.

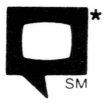

Logo for *VideoCaptions*. Videos bearing this have subtitles, but they will only appear if you have a special machine, called a VideoCaption Reader.

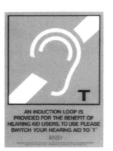

Sign indicating a loop system is installed. To use it, switch the hearing aid to 'T'.

Out and about

Personal amplifiers

These are pocket-sized units which you can carry about for use away from home.

They might be used, for example, at a parents' evening where there are many tables, each with a teacher and two parents talking – hearing aids are not much help when you are surrounded by many different conversations. If you have a personal amplifier with you, you could ask the person speaking to wear a clip-on microphone. You put on the headphones, earphone, ear loop or neck loop provided, and the chosen voice will come straight to your ear.

Some personal amplifiers are fitted with a loop pick-up facility, so that you can use a loop system without a hearing aid.

Loop systems

Many public buildings, like offices, banks, churches and theatres have a loop system installed. Look out for the logo illustrated on the opposite page .

The loop may not cover the whole building; so check that the loop system covers your chosen seat if you are buying tickets for the theatre or cinema.

At the theatre, you may be pleasantly surprised. Theatres are designed with acoustics in mind. The actors are trained to project their voices. Everyone else is quiet. You may hear easily.

Try to arrive several minutes early if you need the loop system. You will then be able to try the 'T' switch before the performance starts and warn a member of staff if it buzzes. Either the system has not been switched on or else it is not working properly.

Some places, like banks and social security offices, have the loop system fitted to certain but not all of their cubicles. Head for one with the loop and the person on the other side will not have to talk about your confidential matters in a raised voice.

Museums, art galleries and the like sometimes supply tapes and headphones for customers to enable them to listen to a commentary as they walk round. Some also provide personal loops or amplifiers for the hard of hearing.

Infra-red systems

These are sometimes used in educational settings so that pupils can hear a teacher speaking from anywhere in the room. No wires are needed – so teacher and pupils can move around freely.

It is also sometimes used in theatres. In this case, you will need head-phones which are usually supplied for a returnable deposit. The 'T' switch does not apply and the sound comes via an invisible infra-red signal. It is picked up by a sensor at the front of the headphones and is fed straight into your ear.

If you put your hand, hanky, or anything in front of the sensor, it will emit a loud buzz and make everybody jump. You will soon stop doing that – but after sitting in a theatre for a couple of hours you may forget. Then an almighty buzz will rock the auditorium when you mop your brow at an emotional moment.

Palantype Computer-Aided Transcripts (CATs)

Computer-aided transcripts are useful in situations where one speaker is addressing a large number of people.

This is a form of instant subtitling. The words appear on a screen almost as soon as they leave the speaker's mouth. This may be an enormous screen readable from the back of a large hall, or a small desk-top version for individuals who are hearing-impaired. It is the next best thing to hearing, if you have good eyesight.

At present there is a shortage of operators with sufficient skill to type at the speed of speech. It cannot be done on an ordinary typewriter but requires a special keyboard on which up to eight keys can be pressed simultaneously. Piano players are at an advantage when learning, as it is similar to playing chords. In fact, the key combinations are called chords.

Words are not typed letter by letter, but sound by sound with many short forms included. Sometimes one chord can represent a whole phrase. That is how such amazing speeds, around 200 words per minute, can be achieved.

There is a computer link between the keyboard and the screen. The computer translates the sound patterns into typed English text. If the operator makes a mistake, the computer will search through its dictionary to find the nearest equivalent – and it usually gets it right. Palantype is around 95% accurate and the remaining 5% is readable. It does not pause. A word takes about one second to journey from the speaker's mouth to the screen.

The system has been used with great success in Parliament, in courts, at police stations, and at meetings attended by large numbers of deaf people. It is worth considering the use of CATs at any large meeting – for an audience of 200 middle-aged people is likely to include about 45 who are hearing-impaired. Many more, who have not yet noticed any loss, will also have some difficulty at a distance.

The equipment and an operator can be hired from Possums Controls Ltd. (see address list). It could make the world of difference.

Prices and availability

Sound Advantage (see address list) maintains a catalogue of assistive devices. You may also be able to obtain them through local organisations for the deaf.

As with any product, prices vary. As a rough guide, at the time of writing, headphones are £5–£12, microphones are £8 and personal listening devices are £30–£60. A domestic loop system is about £80 while infra-red systems start at £200. A phone amplifier is about £25 and a phone flash around £40. Ordinary phones with helpful features are £40–£50 while textphones cost about £280. Door chimes cost £45 and clocks start at about £20.

Chapter 6
Outside Help, Problems at Work
and Public Awareness

Social Services

The Chronically Sick and Disabled Person's Act 1970 obliges local authorities to provide technical aid for long-term sick and disabled people, including the deaf and hard of hearing.

There are no set rules as to what must be provided or for whom – that is left to the discretion of each authority. The only way of finding out what your own authority provides is to ask.

Every local authority has a department of some sort to deal with the hard of hearing – even if the department consists only of one person struggling under a mountain of paper. There is no standard name for the department. It might be called "Deaf Services" or "Sensory Needs" or any of a number of other names. You will have to start by saying what you want in order to get referred to the right person.

The standard procedure is for someone to come to your house to assess your needs. This may take a week or a year – but probably just a few months. The assistance you get will depend on your needs, your circumstances, the policy of the particular local authority and the funds available at the time you apply.

Your application is likely to be favourably received if you are elderly, have other disabilities or are also vulnerable in another way.

An example might be if you live in a remote place and cannot use an ordinary phone. Similarly, you are likely to get what you want if you live in a block of flats and the neighbours have got up a petition because your television is on so loud.

But some authorities have rigid policies. They may have decided never to provide certain equipment in any circumstances. And, in some cases, you may be asked for a contribution.

The Register

Funds for the deaf are desperately low. One reason for this is that the records give a false impression of the level of need. There is a Register maintained by each local authority of deaf and hard of hearing people; but only a small proportion of those who could be on it actually are. In some areas there are over 200 unregistered hearing-impaired people for each one on the Register.

Registration does not happen automatically. You may have been a regular at the ENT clinic for years; but you will not be registered unless you have told the local authority. In the event you move to a different local authority area, you will need to register again.

It is worth getting registered because there are some benefits and assistive devices you can have for the asking – such as a free extension bell for the telephone (from BT). You can also apply to British Rail for a Disabled Person's Railcard, which entitles you to reduced fares for you and a companion.

Even if you do not want anything for yourself, having more names on the Register strengthens the authority's case when it applies for funds. So adding your name to the list might indirectly help someone else with greater need and less money. And you might even be glad of the help yourself one day.

Disability benefits

There are no benefits specifically for the deaf, though deafness is recognised as a qualifying disability.

Depending on your circumstances, you may be able to claim benefits and allowances relating to your disability. Social Services will tell you more about what applies to you; and may liaise with the Benefits Office on your behalf.

Being deaf may make it difficult to communicate your needs and steps are being taken to help with that. All benefit offices now have loop systems; and by the end of 1994, all will have textphones. Many members of staff have learned sign language too. The needs of the deaf really are taken seriously.

Employment

Discrimination

Everyone has the right to be judged on ability rather than disability. This principle is backed up by legislation.

In some instances, employers are required to discriminate positively in favour of the disabled. Any firm or individual who employs twenty or more people must aim to have at least 3% registered disabled on the workforce.

It is not really feasible to enforce that aim in law, for there is no guarantee that disabled people will apply for a particular job – and if they do, they might not be suitable. It is difficult to prove whether an employer's claim that a deaf candidate has "the wrong mix of skills" is genuine or the result of prejudice.

Nevertheless, the law is helpful. Employers sometimes deliberately seek disabled people to make up the quota; and being deaf could tip the balance in your favour. This is another good reason to get yourself registered – even if you dislike the label. Tell yourself that there is nothing degrading about it.

The law also brings the issue of disability at work to the fore by forcing employers to consider people they might otherwise have rejected out of hand. In most cases, they then discover that disabled employees are not liabilities at all. They are as capable, hard-working and reliable as anyone else.

PACTs

PACT stands for Placing Assessment and Counselling Team. Such teams have been set up all over the country. Each consists of a Disability Employment Adviser (DEA) and other experts in the field and will help you in your search for a job – from discussing the options with you to contacting potential employers on your behalf.

They can arrange for a professional communicator to be with you at an interview if you are not able to hear much and have difficulty in communicating. That could be a signer or a lipspeaker (a lipspeaker repeats what is said without using the voice but makes very clear lip patterns and helps by use of facial expression and gesture). Knowing that you will be able to understand what is going on at an interview should help to quell your nerves to the point where you are only just as scared as normally hearing applicants.

Once you are in work, assistive devices can be provided on loan to make things easier. You can also ask for these if you already have a job and your hearing is deteriorating.

Relaxing the rules

It is recognised that having a disability makes looking for a job even tougher than usual. For this reason, some government schemes that normally demand an applicant to have been on the Unemployment Register for three or six months beforehand, relax that rule for the disabled. The schemes to which this applies are Jobsearch, Jobclub, Job Interview Guarantee, and Work Trials.

Jobsearch and Jobclub both offer help in the arduous task of looking and applying for jobs. They also provide you with free access to office facilities.

Job Interview Guarantee, as the name suggests, guarantees that you will have an interview for a job for which you are qualified – so you will get a chance to present yourself.

A Work Trial can sometimes be arranged where you actually do the job for up to three weeks – so that you are able to demonstrate what you can do.

These schemes are designed to get people over the first few hurdles. They are not guarantees of employment but they can provide strong support.

Access to Work

Access to Work is the name of an initiative designed to bring all the varied services offered to the disabled at work – and to their employers – together under one scheme.

Deaf people often object to being thought of as disabled. They shy away from the word "disabled" as though it means "defective". This is really arguing over words. You are at a disadvantage if you have a hearing problem which interferes with your work prospects. It makes no difference whether or not you call that disadvantage a disability.

You do not have to declare yourself disabled to benefit from Access to

Work. It is sufficient to be eligible to go on the Register if you choose to do so.

In the case of deafness, a communicator may be provided together with any assistive device deemed necessary. The rules are flexible, allowing help to be tailored to the needs of the individual and the particular job.

The aim is to promote equal opportunities so that, as far as possible, no one is at a disadvantage in finding a job or advancing in a career.

The Disability Employment Adviser can provide specialist advice and help to employees and employers. Grants can be as high as £21,000 per applicant over five years, after which the process can start again.

Noise at work

Too much noise will make you deaf – there's no doubt about that. It was much less of a problem in days gone by. Ears lasted for far longer when noise at work meant the thud of hooves on soil and the sound of clods of earth being overturned.

But noise-induced deafness occurred even in ancient times. People living near roaring waterfalls could not hear so well as those who had settled beside quiet stretches of water. Today's roaring machinery has the same effect.

Ideally, machines should be made quieter or else put in a soundproof room away from the workers. Failing that, the ears should be protected.

There are laws about this. Employers must provide ear protectors for sound levels as high as 85 decibels – as is likely if there are machines at work. Also they must advise, but need not compel, the workers to wear them.

Employers are obliged to measure and keep a record of the sound level. They cannot get away with saying that they did not know that the noise level was so high.

Measuring sound is complicated. A higher number of decibels means a louder noise – but it is not like measuring with a ruler. 100 decibels is more than twice as loud as 50 decibels – much more!

Whispering makes 50 decibels. 100 decibels is the sound level recorded beside a very busy road – enough to damage the hearing of a traffic warden patrolling there all day every day. Increasing the sound by another 50 decibels to 150, would be as loud as a bomb and could devastate hearing.

You don't need expensive equipment to know when you are at risk. There is a risk if you regularly have to shout to make yourself heard, or if the noise makes your ears ring. If it is like that at work, your employer should be taking steps.

The law is more stringent when sound levels are regularly above 90 decibels, or occasionally above 140 decibels. Workers are then obliged to wear ear protection. They are also obliged to check noise control equipment and to report any faults. The employer must reduce the noise as far as possible; and must provide quiet areas.

It is often difficult to get people to accept safety devices such as ear protection. A survey in the industrial heart of the Midlands found only one group of workers – boilermakers – even willing to consider wearing ear protectors.

Deafness is an occupational hazard for boilermakers. In 1890, a hundred of them were tested and every one was found to have impaired hearing. That does not impress the boilermakers of today for, in the Midlands survey, 84% said "No" to ear protectors.

Some of those men have macho ideals that need challenging. A man is no less of a man because he wants to keep his hearing. "But" goes the argument, "You can't hear anything with those things on". That can be a problem – but it should provide them with some insight into what it is like to be deaf. If they cannot stand it when they can cure it in a couple of seconds by removing the offending muff, how will they cope when the deafness is forever. They won't be so manly then!

Looking at it from another point of view, any claim for compensation will be weaker if ear protectors are provided but not worn.

Types of protectors

There are two types of ear protectors – plugs and muffs.

Plugs go into the ear. They need to be a good fit to be any use. Fingers are a poor fit and do not make good ear plugs. Children realise this when they stuff their fingers in their ears to avoid hearing a telling-off. They still hear it.

The best fitting plugs are made of compressed foam that expands in the ear to make a precise fit. As well as blocking out more noise, they are more comfortable than plastic or rubber ear plugs. There are versions with a hollow channel running through for use if conversation is essential; but remember that if they allow speech, they will allow other noises to come through as well.

Ear muffs are best for intense noise. These are not the furry sort worn in snowy climes, but large pads that cover the entire ear. To work properly they need to fit close to the head. Long hair should be pushed aside for sound waves easily get through any gaps.

Glasses will create big gaps and make the muffs useless. If the person cannot do the job without glasses, or find a way of attaching them after the ear muffs are in place, another person should be sent into the noisy place.

In situations when noise is not the only danger – on building sites where bricks might fall on the head, for example – helmets must be worn. Ear muffs cannot be worn at the same time; but ear plugs can. Ideally, a helmet that incorporates ear protection should be supplied. Even better are helmets with built-in radio communication.

There is no such thing as an ear protector that cuts out all noise. The best earmuffs reduce it by 50 decibels. A quarry worker wearing these when using explosives at 140 decibels, would get 90 decibels – which is still within the danger zone. So he or she would be well advised to have rest periods in quiet places.

The importance of rest from noise

Given a chance, ears can recover from the shock of loud noise – within limits. Lots of people experience dull hearing just after working with power tools, or going on a roller coaster where everybody is screaming. The ears recover after some minutes or hours. They can stand quite a lot. An admiral escaped with his hearing intact after firing 80 broadsides from a cannon. But he was deaf for a whole fortnight immediately afterwards.

Resting the ears between noisy peaks makes a big difference. A shepherd who spends Saturday nights at rock concerts has a week to recover. He is less at risk than a railway porter who works eight hours a day on the underground and spends his evenings doing crossword puzzles. The day in, day out, wear and tear on his inner ear will probably damage his hearing eventually.

Occupational deafness

Occupational deafness is what the DSS calls deafness caused by your job. They have strict definitions about what jobs count and what is meant by deafness; but you can claim benefit if your case falls within those guide-lines.

Details are given in the leaflet "If you think your job has made you deaf" (NI207), obtainable from Social Security offices. It lists nine types of jobs, including forestry, textile manufacturing and dye forging, that involve noisy machinery. To qualify for benefit you must have worked at one of those nine jobs for at least ten years; and you must have left the job sooner than five years ago.

You must also have a hearing loss of at least 50 decibels in each ear; and the loss in at least one ear must have been caused by the job. The DSS states that unless the damage recorded is to the inner ear, it is unlikely to have been caused by too much noise at work.

You will be sent to a Medical Board for a hearing test when you apply and will receive a weekly benefit if the Board concludes that you are at least 20% disabled as a result of noise at work. The greater the disable-ment, the more you will get. You can appeal if you disagree with the decision.

It is also possible to get compensation for tinnitus, although that is far more difficult to measure. There have been some high settlements for this – £50,000 or even more. These cases are very much the exception and the compensation consists mainly of loss of earnings – so there is no real gain.

Public awareness

No-one can help without first being aware of the problem. This creates a dilemma for the deaf person. To tell or not to tell.

Telling means drawing attention to yourself by pointing out a defect. But not telling can be worse. Confusion follows confusion. The longer it goes on, the more embarrassing it gets. Having pretended to hear, it is even more difficult to announce that you are unable to do so.

So lots of people don't tell – which means that other people don't know and it is never discussed. The effect of this is that hearing people do not know how to help, even when they do know that someone is deaf.

Some purveyors of hearing aids capitalise on this embarrassment and talk about "keeping the secret safe". Why should it be a secret? There is noth-ing shameful about it.

You will get no support if you succeed in keeping your disability secret. You will get help if you fail – but only after the misery of being "found out". You will get help straight away if you do not try to hide it. But it is hard to avoid embarrassment altogether for there has to be a moment when you tell.

Some people welcome wearing a conspicuous hearing aid as a way of avoiding saying the words. This presumes that other people will notice. It may seem like a hideous carbuncle to the wearer – surely the first thing that anyone notices? – but actually, people rarely notice at all. If they do, they probably think it is as good as a brand new ear – meaning they have no need to do anything. They will no more make special efforts with their speaking than they would guide someone gently by the elbow because he is wearing glasses.

Badges

Another way is to wear a badge. Organisations for the deaf sell ones that say "Lipreader: please speak clearly", "Hard of hearing: no need to shout", and similar messages. These solve the problem of having to bring up the subject. Talking is one of the best ways to raise awareness; and it is easier to talk about the problem once it has been introduced.

Badges are not the answer to everything. There is a limit to the amount of information you can get into such a small space and people can get the wrong idea. It might be thought that a lipreader will automatically lipread everything, so nothing need be done. If the badge tells them not to shout, they may think "Well, what else can I do?" They may not want to ask questions about it. Hearing people can get embarrassed too.

Badges are an excellent way of providing a small amount of information. At best, they trigger a highly informative debate. They do not suit every-one. For some, the very thought of advertising themselves in this way makes them cringe. If you are one of these, don't even think of wearing one. There's no virtue in it. It is just one of the ways forward – if you like the idea.

Sympathetic Hearing Scheme

There is another idea – in between keeping quiet about it and sporting a badge for all to see. That is using a Sympathetic Hearing Card which can be slipped into a purse or wallet and brought out when required.

The card has the logo for hearing loss (see illustration, page 94) on one side, and suggestions as to how to help on the other. Most people who work with the public are likely to recognise it. If not, reading it will quickly make clear what it is.

This card is the brainchild of Maureen Beaumont, who was plunged into deafness. She wanted people to know about it but found it tiresome explaining to everyone she met.

She hit on the idea of carrying a card that would do her explaining for her. It had to be self-explanatory or she would have to spend even more time explaining what it was about. She needed a logo to represent hearing loss. There was no such thing at the time so her first task was to get one designed and accepted.

This was a big task, especially as no one seemed interested. She plodded on and on, approaching people and writing about it. The trickle of support for her idea slowly increased. The turning point came when Alf Morris, then Minister for the Disabled, took up the idea and asked the four main charities for the deaf to set up a competition to find a good logo.

Competitions unleash talent and some neat designs came up; but they focused on the stereotype of the deaf as helpless. Maureen did not like the winning designs. Nor did the World Federation of the Deaf. In the end, a different logo was adopted (see front cover). This is now a familiar sight on the doors of shops, banks and museums. Walk down any High Street and you will probably see several of them.

Having a well-known logo was a tremendous stride forward. People see it, wonder what it is and ask around to find out. It is a cheap and simple way of getting people to the first stage of awareness – knowing that a problem exists and that things can be done to help.

Awareness-raising courses

The window stickers seen in the High Street are a sign that staff working there are aware of the problems of hearing loss and know how to help.

The Sympathetic Hearing Scheme

 I am deaf/hearing impaired

To enable us to communicate more easily
• Please speak clearly and not too quickly.
• Turn towards the light and face me.
• Cut out as much background noise as possible.
• Don't be afraid to write things down.
• Rephrase rather than repeat. Do not shout.

The British Association of the Hard of Hearing
7–11 Armstrong Road, London, W3 7JL. Telephone: 081 743 1110

The Sympathetic Hearing Card is supplied by "Hearing Concern". They used to be called the "British Association for the Hard of Hearing", as it says on this card. New batches of these cards will bear the name "Hearing Concern".

The stickers are given away after completion of an awareness-raising course. Hearing Concern (see address list) runs these for any organisation that asks for one. They are practical courses, aimed to show how just a modicum of adjustment can make the world of difference.

They use a video that has part of its sound track modified to show what passes for normal with the deaf. This comes as a shock for the hearing who had previously imagined a world of silence. What comes through a hearing aid is a mix-up of every sound around – through which the wearer has to struggle to extract speech. The video shows ordinary situations, like drinking in a pub (difficult because of background noise) and buying a railway ticket (difficult because of the glass partition).

Seeing what a battle it is to do the sort of things the hearing never think twice about, gets people thinking and talking. They remember hard of hearing people they have known and suddenly realise why they seemed so awkward. Often, someone on the course crawls out of the woodwork and admits to having hearing problems. Far from being rebuffed, the sufferer gets rapt attention and understanding.

The time is then ripe for suggestions on how to help. These are simple – even obvious when you think about them. Awareness courses make people think.

People usually remember very well on the day after the course – but memory fades. Hearing Concern provides leaflets that set out the main points. Briefly, these are:

- Don't shout.
- Talk clearly and quite slowly.
- Face the person you are talking to, and face the light.
- Avoid background noise.
- Keep your mouth uncovered.
- Avoid unusual words.
- Re-phrase if necessary, rather than repeating and repeating.
- Be willing to write things down.
- Talk directly to the deaf person and not to a hearing companion. The deaf are not otherwise incompetent.

The last point is important. It is demoralising to be ignored once your disability is discovered. The hearing need to make an effort to include the deaf; and the deaf need to push themselves forward for a two-way communication.

Campaign Charter

There is another side to awareness. Not being able to hear properly makes it more difficult to become aware. We constantly need information like the time of the train and the price of a ticket. It is usually written down somewhere and can be found if we plough through all the leaflets and notices. But it is easier to ask and be told – assuming you can hear, that is.

The RNID has launched a campaign called "Louder than Words" that aims to make information more accessible. They have produced a Campaign Charter of ways to help. There is nothing startling about the suggestions. They are all straightforward ideas that will make the life of a deaf person simpler.

The first point is that the hearing should understand and accept that the deaf have as much right to information as the hearing. The rest follows on from that.

There should be good lighting and not too much background noise – so as to make lipreading easier. If there are glass partitions, they should be made of non-reflective glass for reflections get in the way.

Where possible, equipment like loops and textphones should be provided. This is not a major expense for a large firm. It should not be assumed that, just because an announcement has been made, everybody has heard it. The information should be put on a screen or notice board as well.

There was recently a case reported in which a man was taken to the wrong destination by British Rail. An announcement had been made about the change of route; but as he did not hear it, he just sat on the train until it was obviously wrong. It cost him £25 for a taxi to get to the right place. British Rail did the honourable thing and refunded the taxi fare. It may not be practicable to put a screen on the back of every seat – but it would have been cheaper for British Rail, and more convenient for the passenger, if someone had gone through the train to make sure that everybody knew.

Those who rely on sign language should be able to depend on having a signer available whenever necessary. That is pie in the sky at the moment – but there are a few around. The Benefits Agencies encourage and give financial help to employees who wish to learn to sign. The Halifax Building Society, as another example, is willing to send a signer to your home if you are one of its customers.

Perhaps the greatest help of all is the running of awareness-raising courses. The lives of the deaf would run far more smoothly if everybody were aware of their problems and had some idea of how to help.

Chapter 7
Hearing Dogs

Everybody is familiar with guide dogs for the blind. It is less widely known that there are hearing dogs too.

A dog will help you morning, noon and night. It starts the day by telling you that it is time to get up. When the alarm clock goes, two paws and a nose will appear by your face – or a whole dog, if it is a little one. It will lead you to the right place when the phone rings, when someone is at the door or when the baby cries. It will lead you to the cooker when dinner is ready – it will know by the sound of the timer.

The dog will tell you as soon as it hears the smoke detector if your house catches fire. It will not take you to the fire but will lie down so that you know there is danger and can lead it out of the house.

Dogs are excellent animals for the job. They are sociable creatures that like to please people. It is their nature to listen for unusual sounds. Any dog at all, without training, will rush to the door when someone calls. Training a hearing dog is building on what comes naturally.

The idea of hearing dogs was first launched in this country at Crufts Dog Show in 1982. In amongst all the champion pedigree dogs was a stray from the National Canine Defence League. This was "Favour", destined to become a champion in a different way. Favour, Britain's first demonstration hearing dog, has now retired.

Since then, well over 200 hearing dogs have been trained. Each one has been through weeks or months of socialising and obedience training, followed by what amounts to a rigorous college course for dogs and then given a period of adjustment to life as a fully-fledged hearing dog. 200 dogs represent a lot of hard work – but that number is not sufficient and there is now a waiting list of 18 months.

Sponsorship

Training a hearing dog costs £2,500. The recipients are not asked to pay, though they may want to make a donation.

The money comes from sponsorship. Anyone, or any group of people, can become a sponsor. Some are big business concerns. Others are groups, like the WI, Brownies and a number of schools.

The sponsors get a photograph of the dog, regular progress reports and the choice of its name. They can choose a name to suit their organisation. The Salvation Army, for example, called its dog "Sally Ann".

Selection

A dog has to be good to be chosen. "Good" does not mean a fancy pedigree. It might have one but that is by the way. What matters is that the dog is friendly, willing, intelligent, and neither timid nor too boisterous.

The dog may be any shape or size. Deaf people have the full spectrum of life-styles and a dog that is perfect for one might be wrong for another. A skyscraper-block dweller who reads and does tapestry all day will need a small, placid dog. Someone who goes for regular ten-mile runs will be better off with a larger and more energetic animal.

The dogs are trained for specific individuals – so every applicant gets the right sort of dog. There is no ideal type, nor is any particular breed preferred for training.

Some dogs are gifts from breeders; but most come from rescue centres. Some were bred on puppy farms – the sort of place in which breeding bitches are treated as production machines and used to produce as many litters as biologically possible. The resulting puppies are runts; but with tender, loving care they can thrive and grow up to be highly skilled and much loved assets to their deaf owners. It is a beautiful system of mutual benefit.

Socialisers

Dogs are not expected to go straight from their mothers into intensive training. The first few weeks or months are spent at the home of a volunteer called a socialiser. The job of the socialiser is to get the dog up to good pet standard. It lives at home as a family pet and gets used to the general hurly-burly of life in the house and out and about.

A hearing dog is expected to go anywhere the owner wants to go – so it must be happy in all sorts of places. One that cringes when lorries come past will be a nuisance when walking along busy roads. It is the socialiser's job to get the dog used to traffic, railway stations, shopping centres, fields of sheep and as many different places as possible.

The dog must also be reliable when meeting people, especially children who may want to cart it around. So it is introduced to lots of different people on its travels.

If there are no children in the socialiser's house, it will be taken to visit schools. That is an education for the children too. They learn about deafness, the problems it causes and how a dog can help.

Alongside this, the dog must be up to scratch in basic obedience. Every month the dogs gather at a "puppy playgroup" held at the training centre. These are fun sessions with serious intent. They play doggy games that involve the dog sitting or coming, walking to heel or whatever it is told to do. The dog gets a reward when it gets it right, with plenty of praise – tails wag all round!

Training is made fun because that is the best way to learn. There is nothing haphazard about it. The dog is working towards a goal; and it takes regular progress tests on its way to gaining its three certificates in obedience.

It is a tribute to the work of the socialisers that most dogs reach such high standards. The pass rate is at least as good as for guide dogs for the blind – and those dogs are specially bred for the purpose. Hearing dogs mostly start out as rescued puppies.

Some dogs do fail though and become "rejects". That sounds dreadful; but a rejected dog is still likely to be a very good dog indeed – but one that has not quite made the grade.

The training centre at the organisation, Hearing Dogs for the Deaf, has a list of people willing to provide good homes. Let them know if you would like to go on the list (see address list).

Becoming a socialiser

You may be interested in becoming a socialiser. You could still become a week-end socialiser even if you work and cannot take in a dog full time. The dogs are kept in kennels during training and it is good for them to have a week-end break with some more socialising experience.

The job is unpaid; but a contribution is made towards feeding and travel expenses. Essential equipment is provided and the vet's bills are covered in full. You will get plenty of support from the Puppy Supervisor and a free book (on loan for as long as you remain a socialiser) that tells you the ins and outs of caring for and socialising dogs.

This is a rewarding, demanding, and essential job. If you think you can do it, then let them know at the training centre. They will be glad to hear from you.

Training

Ready for training

The dog will come back to the kennels when it is ready.

The waiting list is studied to see which deaf person this dog is most likely to suit. It is not a strict first-come, first-served system for there is no point in having a dog sooner if it is the wrong sort of dog for you.

When a suitable dog is found, the recipient is sent a photograph and an invitation to visit the kennels. Getting to meet the dog is a big boost to morale after a typical wait of around eighteen months. Taking it for a walk and calling it by name is quite different from receiving a dry letter confirming eligibility.

The count-down to D-Day, the day the dog comes home, can begin – although it is still four months away.

Training begins

The dog then starts "college". This is a furnished house in which it will learn and practise hearing skills.

The college consists of two houses, each like a semi-detached bungalow with a bedroom in its loft. They were built from the shell of a building-site cabin, specially donated for the purpose.

Each house has three doorbells. Which one is used depends on the sort of bell in the dog's future home. The doors are different too. One house has a glazed door and the other a solid one. The dog is trained in the one with the same sort of door as its future home. This matters to the dog, because of what it sees, or does not see, when a visitor calls. It can see the shape of a person through a glazed door, but not through a solid one. If that changes when the dog actually begins its duties, it could get confused.

The alarm clock used is the same for all the dogs. A similar clock is given to the deaf person when the dog goes home – so there is no change there.

The dog goes to college for lessons every day. First it must learn to respond to a squeaker. When the squeaker goes, the dog must stop whatever it is doing and go and put a paw on the trainer's leg. For this it gets rewarded with a treat of some kind. It might be a titbit, a rub-tummy or a game of ball. It does not matter what the reward is, so as long as the dog likes it.

Reward is vital. Punishment is pointless; and, apart from being unkind, it does not work. Imagine trying to learn something and being hit with a rolled up newspaper every time you make a mistake. Punishment does not work for people or for dogs.

The dog is taught other noises, like the doorbell and the phone, as soon as it has learned to respond reliably to the squeaker. It is taught to come and put a paw on the trainer's leg when it hears the noise. The trainer asks "What is it?" and the dog must then lead the way to the door, the phone or whatever. Later on, it is taught a hand signal as well – so speech is not essential.

The dog also helps when a deaf person does not hear someone call. When someone says "Fetch Mummy", the dog will go to find Mummy. It places a paw on her leg and then takes her to whoever was calling. In most households, Mummy is the one who is called most often – but other names can be substituted.

The dog's socialisation continues while this training is going on. It goes on expeditions into town and elsewhere, so as not to forget ordinary life. And obedience training also continues.

Getting to know each other

It takes four months for a dog to learn all the necessary skills. By that time it has become very fond of the trainer.

Fortunately, dogs transfer their affections reasonably easily; but they cannot just be despatched to the homes of recipients and left to get on with it. The recipient, too, has some learning to do.

So the recipient comes to stay in a flat at the training centre. Dog and recipient then work together, practising hearing skills in the training house and also going for walks, for trips into town. They generally get to know each other.

After five days, the recipient takes the dog home; and they are both left to settle down quietly together for several more days before the next stage.

Follow-up

It is best for any problems to be discovered and put right as soon as possible.

Big problems are rare but there are sometimes little niggles to be sorted out. Perhaps the dog is pining and cries at night. Perhaps it is not eating as well as the recipient would like.

The Placement Counsellor will make a routine visit, staying somewhere in the locality for three days, during which any worries can be sorted out and practicalities like registering with a vet are done. If the dog is going to work with the recipient, the Counsellor will also visit the workplace. If there are people there who are unhappy about having a dog on the premises, the Counsellor will talk to them.

After that, daily reports are sent to the training centre for a month. Then there is a check-up visit to ensure that the dog and recipient are happy together. The training centre is only a phone call away if any problems should arise.

Triumph

The dog is given its final assessment after it has been in its new home for three months. If it passes, it gets a certificate with a photograph. It will wear the garb of honour – a yellow coat, collar and lead – and its name will appear in the next edition of the Hearing Dogs Newsletter.

As a fully qualified hearing dog, it will be entitled to free veterinary treatment, to complimentary insurance from Pet Protect, to cheap food from Pedigree Petfoods and to some free transport by bus, train and plane.

At present, guide dogs for the blind enjoy more concessions and are allowed in more places than hearing dogs. But it may be assumed that, as awareness grows, hearing dogs will be afforded the same status.

How do you get a hearing dog?

It is estimated that 85 out of 1000 people could benefit from a hearing dog. There are not nearly enough dogs to go round; but the situation should improve soon when a second training centre is opened. Meanwhile, there is a long waiting list. Contact Hearing Dogs for the Deaf (see address list) if you want your name to be added to it.

To qualify, you must be severely deaf, or worse, and have no one at home to help for much of the time. You must genuinely want a dog and not just think it would be useful. Hearing dogs are not pets as such; but they are as sociable and affectionate as any other dog and it would be unfair to treat them as just another device.

People with other disabilities as well as deafness can apply for a hearing dog if they think that is their greatest need. They might prefer a guide dog, or a dog trained to carry things to the wheelchair. They cannot have a team of dogs; and hearing dogs are normally only given to households that have no other dog – though an exception might be made in the case of an elderly pet.

What if you don't qualify?

There is nothing to stop you teaching your own dog a few tricks if you are not deaf enough to need everything a hearing dog has to offer, but could do with a bit of extra help. The dog will not reach anything like the standard of a professionally trained animal – but every little helps.

There are obedience classes all over the country and these may be located by asking at a pet shop or the library. It is a good idea to have an obedient dog in any case; and the person in charge should at least be able to give advice about training.

It is easy enough to teach a dog to tell you there is someone at the door. You will probably know anyway, even without hearing the barks, if you are in the same room. The dog will suddenly get up and run to the door. If you can teach it to come to you first, you will always know.

This is easy if the dog comes when it is called. If it does not, go to more obedience classes. Then, when the doorbell rings and the dog rushes off, call it back. Give it a reward, take it with you to the door and reward it again. If you repeat that often enough, the dog will automatically come to you first.

It will be quicker for you to organise your own training sessions, rather than wait for the bell to ring – especially if you may not hear it and so sometimes take no notice. Practise by getting a willing friend to ring the bell. Let the friend in and out again.

Let him or her ring again a minute or so later.

Do not do this for too long – partly for the sake of your friend but for the dog as well. Dogs, like people, get bored; and boredom is a barrier to learning.

Be ready with the reward. Dogs only remember for a few seconds and a reward given minutes later will be meaningless. Once the dog has learned well, you need not give a reward every single time – but keep the praise flowing.

Be patient if the dog does not seem to be learning. Give up the idea, at least for the time being, if you find yourself getting cross.

Don't punish the dog. If you do, it will go off the idea and start slinking away. Its learning will slow down or stop. It will not understand – it will associate punishment with the general situation but will not have a clue why you suddenly turned nasty. It is far better just to stop.

If the dog learns the idea of answering the door, you can then try using the same principle for the phone, the alarm clock and whatever else you choose.

Repetition, little and often, with lots of praise – and no harsh words – will sooner or later teach most dogs to come to you when they hear a particular noise. Good luck!

Chapter 8
Deafness and the Ear

How the ear works (when it does work)

Sound waves travel through the air at about 765 miles an hour. They pass through the ear where they are turned into electrical impulses. These are transmitted to the brain, which in turn translates them into words, music, and so on.

A total number of about 350,000 different sounds can be distinguished by the brain; and the whole process takes about 30 milliseconds.

Outer ear

The first port of call is the outer ear – the bit you can see – but this only plays a small part. It simply serves as a funnel to pass the sound waves through to the next stage.

The external auditory canal, or ear hole, leads from the outer ear to the middle ear.

Middle ear

The ear drum is situated at the entrance to the middle ear. This is about as thick as a single sheet of newspaper. It vibrates rapidly in response to sound, moving by a minute amount – only a billionth of a centimetre at some frequencies.

The vibrations then travel through the middle ear along three tiny bones, called the hammer, the anvil and the stirrup because of their shapes.

These are the smallest bones in the body, all three together measuring only about 16mm in length. They form an intricate lever system which propels the sound waves through an opening, called the oval window, into the inner ear.

Inner ear

The sound waves travel on – now through fluid – round a snail-shaped organ called the cochlea, which contains thousands of microscopic hairs.

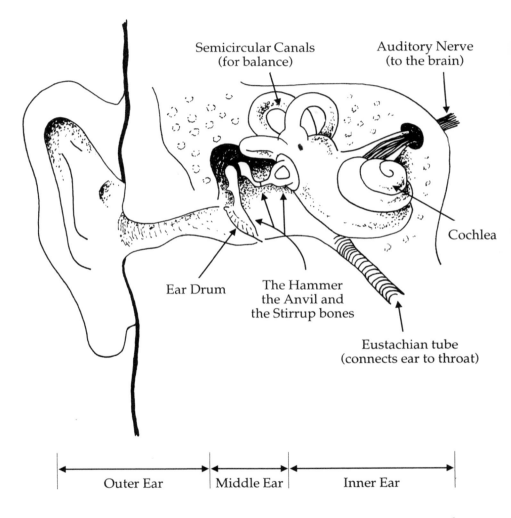

Semicircular Canals
(for balance)

Auditory Nerve
(to the brain)

Cochlea

Ear Drum

The Hammer
the Anvil and
the Stirrup bones

Eustachian tube
(connects ear to throat)

Outer Ear | Middle Ear | Inner Ear

THE EAR

The sound waves cause ripples in the fluid; and the ripples in turn disturb the hairs.

These hairs have been compared to the strings of the harp. A different frequency is registered, depending on which hairs are disturbed – or which strings plucked.

The movement of the hairs triggers electrical impulses which are sent down the auditory nerve to the brain, where they are decoded.

And so we hear.

Types of deafness

Conductive deafness

Deafness resulting from problems in the middle ear is called conductive, or obstructive, deafness.

This means that something prevents the sound waves from being efficiently conducted to the inner ear.

Perceptive deafness

It is in the inner ear that the process of the perception of sound (as opposed to the passive receiving of it) begins.

So problems in the inner ear are referred to as perceptive deafness. Other terms used are sensorineural deafness and nerve deafness.

Prognosis

Broadly speaking, the deeper inside the ear the problem lies, the less chance there is of successful treatment. Excess wax in the outer ear can be quickly syringed away. Inner ear damage is mostly irreversible – though work is being done and there is now some hope.

It is possible to have more than one type of deafness at the same time. If you get worse after being told that you will not, the additional deafness may have another cause. It is worth going back to the doctor to ask.

Causes of deafness

Wax

Wax is produced by all healthy ears. This starts out as white droplets which accumulate with time and become brown and sticky.

Wax may not be pleasant to see; but it should be regarded as a friend of the ear. It helps to prevent dust and moisture from penetrating deep inside the ear and also contains complex chemicals – enzymes and immunoglobulins – to fight infection.

Despite this, wax is often treated like dirt. Cotton buds, bits of tissue and even paper clips are twirled round as deeply as they will go. This rough treatment can make abrasions; and these provide a cosy home for infections, which have more chance of making trouble when the protective wax has been removed. The ear compensates by producing extra wax – so there is really no point in trying to get rid of it.

Some people do produce too much wax. One survey suggested that this is a problem for one person in eight. In such cases, the wax level builds up slowly and is not noticed. Then one day, after a bath or a swim, water gets in to the ear, making the wax swell so as to block the ear canal completely. Hey presto – that person is deaf.

It is a mild form of deafness that seems bad because it occurred so suddenly. The cure is equally sudden – the ears are syringed and the patient hears again.

Infections

When germs infect the ear, the membrane lining to the outer or middle ear becomes painful and inflamed. Pus is produced.

Infections of the outer ear may be caused by incidents such as swimming in dirty water, implements used to remove wax, or eczema possibly aggravated by scratching. In themselves they cause little, if any, deafness.

Infections can get to the middle ear through a tube, called the Eustachian tube, that goes from the back of the throat to the middle ear and provides an easy route for bacteria in the throat. Scarlet fever, measles, the common cold, or any respiratory infection might affect the middle ear and create pus there. Unless this is treated, it can cause deafness by clogging up the bones inside the ear.

This was once the commonest cause of hearing impairment in children; but it is rapidly cured today. Intense pain sends people scurrying to the doctor without delay. And antibiotics will usually reduce the bacteria to a painless level within a few days.

Glue ear

The miracle of antibiotics has not solved all the problems though. Once the pain has gone, many people consider themselves cured and stop taking the medicine. But it takes several more days of treatment to destroy all traces of the bacteria.

Pus from an infection can remain in the ear, even after the death of the bacteria. It creates new problems there because old pus thickens in time to the consistency of glue. Unless treated, this will eventually cause deafness. This is not the only cause of glue ear; but it may be the reason why the number of reported cases has increased in the last few decades.

The standard treatment today is for a grommet – a tiny tube that serves as a drainage hole – to be inserted in the ear. This prevents the build-up of pus by allowing fluid to drain away.

The grommet, a foreign body, is eventually ejected by the ear – usually without even being noticed. It then may or may not be necessary to insert another one.

Otosclerosis

Otosclerosis is the commonest form of hearing loss experienced before the onset of middle age.

The word means hardening of the earbones – a surprising name in a way, because the bones actually go soft and spongy. What happens can be compared to pouring mud over a mechanism that relies on fine movement. It will no longer budge and so becomes hard in the sense of rigid.

The stirrup, the last bone of the three in the chain, becomes firmly fixed in the oval window leading to the inner ear. It blocks the sound waves, instead of pushing them forward.

Victorian doctors knew what needed doing – the bones had to be released by surgery. They managed to open up the ear and perform that operation, thereby improving the hearing. But before the days of antibiotics, infection invariably followed and the technique had to be abandoned.

Surgeons then had the idea of opening up a window to the inner ear to enable more sound to get through. This worked up to a point. Hearing improved – but there were unpleasant side effects like dizziness. Patients had to be forbidden ever to get water in their ears again. So swimming was forbidden and washing the hair became a risky enterprise. This operation continued to be performed until the 1950's.

In 1952 an alternative was discovered by accident. A surgeon, just about to start making the window, accidentally knocked against the stirrup and dislodged it. As luck would have it, the patient was only under local anaesthetic. He exclaimed with amazement that he could hear all of a sudden – and before the operation had properly begun.

Since then, the idea has been developed. The stirrup bone is now removed and a false one inserted in its place. This operation is called a stapedectomy. It succeeds in improving the hearing of over 90% of patients.

Noise-induced deafness

The world is a far noisier place than it was. We travel to work against a background of motor engines and the constant clack, clack, clack of trains. There is a steady throb of machinery when we get there – even in offices. Washing machines, vacuum cleaners, televisions and music systems assail our hearing in the home. Ears were designed for a quieter life.

Eyes are dazzled when exposed to too much light. The eyelids instantly screw up to protect the retina. But there are no earlids to clamp down on the ears to shut out excessive sound.

Some limited protection is provided by tiny muscles inside the ears. These react in response to sudden loud noise, like that from a door slamming, and restrict the volume of noise getting through to the inner ear. But the muscles tire quickly and stop working altogether if the noise goes on and on. Continuous loud noise is a real problem. That's why there are laws about it (see chapter 6).

Accidents

A blow to the head can disrupt any part of the ear.

The small bones of the middle ear may break. It is now possible to see inside the middle ear with a binocular microscope and to repair such fractures.

Damage to the inner ear may not show up on an X-ray. There is probably a microscopic injury if deafness persists for six months after a head injury, even if the X-ray shows no fracture.

Deafness following concussion often disappears after a few days or weeks.

Menière's Disease

Menière's Disease is a disorder of the organ of balance within the inner ear.

Patients experience deafness, tinnitus (ringing in the ears) and vertigo. Vertigo, in this context, means the sensation that the world is spinning around – such as some people get when looking over a precipice. They may or may not be afraid of heights.

This can happen anywhere and at any time. Sufferers stagger and cling on to things for support; or they may drop to the ground and stay there. They feel sick and will probably vomit, though there is nothing wrong with their stomachs. The sensation experienced has much the same characteristics as seasickness. It feels like being in a small boat on a stormy sea.

All this sensation is accompanied by thundering tinnitus and a feeling of puffiness inside the ear. It continues for anything from a few minutes to several hours.

People suffering their first attack can be excused for thinking they are about to die. In fact Menière's Disease is not life-threatening, though there is a risk of accident if the sense of balance suddenly disappears. It is wise to take suitable precautions, like not standing closer than six feet from the edge of a railway platform.

The good news is that there are long remissions, months or years, during which there are no symptoms at all. Some say that the disease burns itself out; but it is hard to know whether it has, since the symptoms may return at any time.

Deafness associated with Menière's Disease

With Menière's, the hearing fluctuates. It may be near normal on good days and drop off again. The trend, however, is slowly but steadily downwards.

Most patients are only affected in one ear. This means that vertigo is the main problem, as the unaffected ear hears perfectly well.

For about one patient in twenty, the second ear follows suit. Then deafness is likely to be the main problem, as the vertigo can generally be controlled by taking tablets.

Where this does not work, an operation may be considered. This should not be undertaken lightly though, for there is a high risk of losing the hearing altogether as a result. The vertigo has to be extremely serious before such a drastic solution is ever adopted.

Presbyacusis

Presbyacusis is the term for the deafness of old age. It is not inevitable and there are octogenarians who hear well – but most do not. The incidence of hearing loss rises from 1 in 56 in the 17-30 age group, to 2 in 3 of those over 80.

The deafness of old age is perceptive deafness, originating in the inner ear. Decades of stimulation of the hairs of the cochlea cause general wear and tear, resulting in deterioration of the hearing.

There is likely to be more presbyacusis around as time goes on and people live longer and longer in a noisier world – that is, unless a cure can be found. There is now some hope.

Can deafness be cured? Hopes for the future

Two hundred years ago, a doctor remarked that there were two kinds of deafness – that caused by wax which was curable, and that caused by anything else which was not.

He would be startled and excited to see present day developments. We do not have to wait for another two hundred years to see even greater differences. Ten years should suffice!

Cochlear implants

The cochlea, deep inside the ear, converts sound waves into electrical impulses which are then transmitted to the brain, where they are decoded into sounds we can understand.

Most deafness results from damage in this area. A cochlear implant may be considered where the damage is bad enough to cause profound deafness.

The operation consists of implanting electrodes to take over the job normally done by the cells of the cochlea – sending impulses to the brain. The electrodes do not do the task nearly so well; but they do permit most patients to hear a little and so facilitate lipreading. In very successful cases, patients may be able to understand speech without lipreading and even use the telephone.

Experiments are now being carried out in London to refine the operation. The aim is to achieve a better result by goading more nerve fibres into action, as well as making the procedure less of a shock to the patient.

A new material called Bioglass is also being tried out to bond other materials to skin and bone. If all goes well, Bioglass will be used to house the components that connect the electrodes within the ear to the speech processor outside. This could mean the replacement of the bulky body-worn speech processors needed at present by small ear-level devices – which would be a great boost to morale.

Can the cochlea be mended?

Sound waves must be converted into electrical impulses to be heard; and this is the job of the nerve cells in the cochlea. These nerve cells do not work properly in four cases out of five of deafness.

Scientists are now no longer so sure that nothing can be done to repair these damaged cells. There has been no single spectacular discovery, but rather a steady flow of little oddments of useful information. When all these are put together, some hope emerges that a cure – even for profound deafness – will come in the end.

The first surprise was the discovery that the nerve cells of fish can sometimes heal themselves. Then it was found that deaf chickens sometimes regain their hearing, with new nerve cells taking over from the ones that have died. This may be a pointer to human cell behaviour too.

Guinea pigs, being bright little animals, can be trained to respond to hearing tests in much the same way as do humans. In such tests, guinea pigs have re-grown damaged balance cells – which are close to hearing cells. Human balance cells have also re-grown – but so far only in a test tube.

In yet another project, hearing cells from the embryo of a rat were made to re-grow in a test tube. All this seems a long way from treating living human ears; but they are all steps in the right direction. Scientists are cautious by nature, unlike journalists who thrive on extravagant claims. So when scientists say "Preliminary tests suggest that these findings may be of some benefit to some patients in certain circumstances", it is a hopeful sign.

Tales of miracles should be taken with a pinch of salt, but scientists do now say that there is cause for optimism. Even if it takes several decades – and it should be quicker than that – today's children may be spared from the deafness of old age.

The advances of the last few years have been faster than anyone predicted.

The possibility of a cure for inner-ear deafness is now somewhere between science fiction and a promise.

Hearing aids

Hearing aids have been around for the past hundred years. The first clumsy boxes, that simply made everything louder, were hailed as a breakthrough at the time.

Research then concentrated on making them smaller. Some aids are now so small that some people fear they might fall into the inner ear and get lost – though that cannot happen.

Apart from size, hearing aids remained much the same for decades. They could only turn up or turn down the volume of sound; and made no allowance at all for different types of hearing loss.

The normal human ear is a highly sophisticated organ. Efforts are now being made to mimic the way it performs.

Automatic gain control

The ear has the natural ability to make adjustments according to the noise level around it. Loud sounds are played down; and quiet sounds played up.

Hearing aids are available that will do this up to a point; but more sophisticated ones are on the way. Researchers at Cambridge University have produced a prototype that detects when the noise level is increasing and automatically turns down the volume of sound. It turns the volume back up again as soon as things become quiet.

So at a party, the volume would be high at first when only a few guests are standing around. It would then decrease as the party becomes rowdy and the music louder. In the car on the way home, the volume would be turned up again.

All this happens without touching the hearing aid. Anyone who has struggled with the volume control of a normal aid – up, down, up, down – and alternately has been blasted out, or shunted into silence, will know what a relief that would be.

Also, the prototype can adjust the volume as quick as a wink. A sudden shriek or the sound of a door slamming makes it switch off and immediately back on again – so nothing is missed except the pain that would have been caused by the loud noise.

Frequency selectivity

High frequency sounds are usually the first to be lost – so most deaf people would benefit from a hearing aid that boosts the high frequency sounds more than those of low frequency. It is the other way round in some cases; but is comparatively rare for both low and high frequencies to be lost in equal measure.

Some existing hearing aids boost some frequencies at the expense of others; but the Cambridge researchers are working on better ways of doing it by the use of digital signal processing.

Digital processing is based on computer programmes rather than on complex circuitry, and uses digital chips. Amazing advances have already been made in this work.

However, there is still much to be done; and producing a wearable hearing aid is another thing from building a prototype in the laboratory. The hope is that aids will be custom-built for each individual in the future.

If this happens, wearing a hearing aid will become less like being attached to a noise machine and more like having your ears back again. Then more people will wear hearing aids and it may be possible to forget that you are deaf – just as people with glasses can forget they are short-sighted.

A final word

Adding the distant possibility of an actual cure to these future advances in hearing aids, it could be that debilitating deafness will be consigned to the history books one day. We can all hope!

Useful Addresses

Association of Teachers of Lipreading to Adults (ATLA)
c/o The Post Office, Slimbridge, Gloucestershire GL2 7BL.

Benefit Enquiry Line
Phone: 0800 882200. Minicom: 0800 243355.

Breakthrough Deaf-Hearing Integration
Charles Gillet Centre, Selly Oak College
Birmingham B29 6LE.
Phone: 021 472 6447. Minicom: 021 471 1001.

British Deaf Association
38 Victoria Place, Carlisle, Cumbria CA1 1HU.
Phone/Minicom: 0228 48844.

British Deaf Sports Council
7a Bridge Street, Otley, West Yorks LS21 1BQ.
Phone: 0943 850214. Minicom: 0943 850081.

British Tinnitus Association
Room 6, 14-18 West Bar Green, Sheffield SD1 2DA.
Phone: 0742 796600.

BT Action for Disabled Customers
Room B4036, BT Centre, 81 Newgate Street,
London EC1A 7AJ.
Phone: 0345 581456.

Council for the Advancement of Communication with Deaf People
Pelaw House, School of Education, University of Durham,
Durham DH1 1TA.
Phone/Minicom: 091 374 3607.

Deaf Broadcasting Council
70 Brackettswood Drive, Chorleywood
Ricksmansworth, Herts WD3 5QQ.

Friends for the Young Deaf Trust
East Court Mansions, College Lane,
East Grinstead RH19 3LT.
Phone: 0342 323444. Minicom: 0342 312639.

Hearing Aid Council
Witan Court, 305 Upper Fourth Street
Central Milton Keynes MK9 1EH.
Phone: 0908 585442.

Hearing Concern
7-11 Armstrong Road, London W3 7JL.
Phone/Minicom: 081 743 1110.

Hearing Dogs for the Deaf
Training Centre, London Road,
Lewknor, Oxford OX9 5RY.
Phone/Minicom: 0844 353898.

Hearing Research Trust
330-332 Grays Inn Road, London WC1X 8EE.
Phone: 071 833 1733.

Menière's Society
Maybury Road, Woking, Surrey GU21 5HX.
Phone: 0483 740597.

National Association of Deafened People
103 Heath Road, Widnes, Cheshire WA8 7NU.
Phone/Minicom: 051 424 3977.

National Centre for Cued Speech
29-30 Watling Street, Canterbury, Kent CT1 2UD.
Phone/Minicom: 0227 450757.

National Deaf Children's Society
45 Hereford Road, London W2 5AH.
Phone/Minicom: 071 229 9272.

Possum Controls Ltd
8 Farmbrough Close, Aylesbury Vale Industrial Park,
Stocklake, Aylesbury, Bucks HP20 1DQ.
Phone: 0296 81591.

Royal Association in Aid of Deaf People (RAD)
27 Old Oak Road, London W3 7HN.
Phone/Minicom: 081 743 6187.

Royal National Institute for Deaf People (RNID)
105 Gower Street, London WC1E 6AH.
Phone: 071 383 3154. Minicom: 071 388 6038.

Sound Advantage
1 Metro Centre, Welbeck Way, Peterborough PE2 7UH.
Phone: 0733 361199. Minicom: 0733 238020.

Sympathetic Hearing Scheme
7-11 Armstrong Road, London W3 7JL.
Phone: 081 740 4447.

Tinnitus Helpline
Phone/Minicom: 0345 090210.

Typetalk
Pauline Ashley House, Ravenside Retail Park,
Speke Road, Liverpool L24 8QB.
Phone: 051 494 1000. Minicom: 051 494 1085.

A selection of other titles from Imperia Books

You Can Beat Arthritis

"This is an excellent book – and much overdue. It should have a place on the bookshelf in every home." *Dr Ann Robinson*

Too many people put up with the pain of arthritis unaware of the options now available to them. This book explains all the medical and alternative remedies successful in treating arthritis, rheumatism and related back pain.

The book provides fresh insight into the conditions which aggravate arthritis, explains how these can be remedied and reveals the key to a greatly improved quality of life. The message throughout the book is one of hope.

Price £11.95 inclusive of postage and handling

£500 A Week From Car Boot Sales

This insider's guide tells all there is to know about successful car booting. It lifts the lid off the booting phenomenon and exposes the massive profits being made weekly in the big money spinner of the 1990s.

The book reveals how to obtain stock for next to nothing, how to find the best pitches and sell at 1000% profit. It also shows how to turn browsers into buyers and discloses ways of telling real antiques from junk.

Buyers, novice booters and even experienced sellers will be amazed by Roger Morgan's account of all the tricks of the trade – the cons, the frauds, the fakes and the selling and buying ploys one would never even dream of.

Price £9.95 inclusive of postage and handling

1,717 Natural Healing Remedies (Kulopathy)

This book reveals many vital remedies based on natural and alternative medicines. It also tells how to detect and overcome the nutritional deficiencies which cause bad health.

Here is just a small selection of the many remedies contained in the book:

8 ways to combat arthritis • 6 remedies for incontinence and other bladder problems • 4 treatments for prostate disorders • 3 ways to reduce breathlessness • 4 ways of overcoming impotence • 3 suggestions to lower blood pressure • A simple treatment to relieve piles • 4 remedies for bad indigestion • 7 suggestions for poor sleepers

Price £9.95 inclusive of postage and handling

How To Find Your Ideal Partner

This book is for the millions of unattached people, whether single, divorced or widowed, who hope one day to form a close loving relationship with an ideal partner.

Readers are shown how to develop a greater understanding of themselves and the type of partner they are seeking. Many different methods of meeting a potential partner are explored – from leisure activities to introduction agencies, from singles clubs to personal ads.

The author also gives helpful, practical advice on how to create the right impression and build a relationship from the first date to a long term commitment.

Price £9.95 inclusive of postage and handling

Quest For The Messiah

This book tells the fascinating story of Man's constant struggle to create a paradise on earth.

Throughout history, self-professed messiahs arose again and again in response to biblical prophesies whenever human suffering reached a new peak. These ranged from saints and pious simpletons to megalomaniac tricksters. The terrible struggles of their followers from the time of Jesus to the present day makes fascinating reading.

Scrupulously researched, Quest for the Messiah is the story of the highest human aspirations and the curious mixture of genuine piety, sex, violence and sheer evil that so often resulted. It is an enthralling story – and a true one!

Price £9.95 inclusive of postage and handling

To order any of the above books, please send your name, address, book titles required and payment (cheque/P.O. or Visa/Access number and expiry date) to Imperia Books Limited, P O Box 191, Edgware, Middlesex HA8 7NY.

Please allow 7 to 21 days for delivery. A full refund will be given for books returned within 28 days.